Getting Past the Affair

To my dear Friend, Bob.
Working with you was a
transformational experience for me.
Words cannot adequately
express the depth of my
admiration and appreciation
of you.
— Doug

Getting Past the Affair

A Program to Help You Cope, Heal, and Move On—Together or Apart

Douglas K. Snyder
Donald H. Baucom
Kristina Coop Gordon

THE GUILFORD PRESS
New York / London

A Division of Guilford Publications, Inc.
72 Spring Street, New York, NY 10012
www.guilford.com

The information in this volume is not intended as a substitute for consultation
with healthcare professionals. Each individual's health concerns should be
evaluated by a qualified professional.

Printed in the United States of America

This book is printed on acid-free paper.

Last digit is print number: 9   8   7   6   5   4   3   2   1

Library of Congress Cataloging-in-Publication Data

Snyder, Douglas K.
    Getting past the affair: a program to help you cope, heal, and move on—
together or apart / Douglas K. Snyder, Donald H. Baucom, Kristina Coop
Gordon.
        p.   cm.
    Includes bibliographical references and index.
    ISBN-13: 978-1-57230-801-5 — ISBN-10: 1-57230-801-X (pbk.: alk. paper)
    ISBN-13: 978-1-59385-357-0 — ISBN-10: 1-59385-357-2 (cloth: alk. paper)
    1. Marital psychotherapy.   2. Adultery—Psychological aspects.
    I. Baucom, Donald H.   II. Gordon, Kristina Coop.   III. Title.
    RC488.5.S627 2006
    616.89′1562—dc22

                                                                2006017066

The case illustrations in this book are based on the authors' research and
clinical practice. In all instances, names and identifying information have been
changed.

*To all the couples who shared with us their
intimate struggles of recovery from an affair.
Your testimonies of trial and triumph bear witness
to the healing potential of love, commitment,
and hard work.*

Contents

Contents

Part III. Can This Marriage Be Saved?

Acknowledgments

This book evolved from years of clinical practice, our own empirical research, and discussions with trusted colleagues about the best means of helping couples struggling to recover from an affair. Along the way several people provided special encouragement and assistance facilitating completion of this work.

We thank our editors at The Guilford Press—especially Kitty Moore, whose steadfast encouragement and patience never wavered despite the passing of numerous deadlines. Kitty and her colleagues—Chris Benton and Sarah Lavender Smith—provided keen insights following an initial draft of the manuscript, and Chris's exquisite attention to editing of the text was invaluable. We also thank Anna Brackett for her care during the final stages of production.

The support and encouragement of our colleagues, students, and clients have been vital. Our thinking was frequently sharpened by lively discussions about relationship injuries, forgiveness, and strategies for promoting recovery. Our clients consistently affirmed the goal of offering these strategies in a manner that couples could pursue on their own. Our dedication of this book to our couples reflects both our admiration and our indebtedness for all they have shared with us.

Above all, we are profoundly grateful for the faithful encouragement of our spouses—Linda Snyder, Linda Baucom, and Andrew Gordon— without whom we could not have completed this book. Your understanding and loving support throughout this project sustained and strengthened us during times we needed it most. Thank you for sharing with us the best of what marriage can offer.

Introduction

Susan sat motionless in front of the computer. She didn't know how long she'd been there and just stared at the screen in disbelief. "I can't wait to be with you again. Last time was incredible—I still can't find my bra!" Someone named Gina had written those words to her husband.

She had been searching for a friend's address when she discovered a series of e-mails to Michael with sexually suggestive subject lines.

Susan could hardly absorb what she'd read. Her brain had turned off and she felt numb. In one brief moment, her life had changed forever. She felt utterly destroyed.

If you've discovered that your partner has had an affair, you probably know how Susan feels. Waves of painful emotion can make it hard to put one foot in front of the other and just go about your daily business. The barrage of conflicting thoughts about how this could have happened—and the haunting flashbacks and questions about what actually did happen—may be so distracting that you can't get anything done. And when you even think about how you're *supposed* to react as the woman scorned or the betrayed man, the only solutions that come to mind are the types of soap opera clichés you've always laughed at. So what *are* you supposed to do?

We wrote this book to walk you through an agonizing time in your life and lead you to the answer that's best for you. The best answer for you may not prove to be the best answer for your partner—and certainly not for the couple down the street. But each of you has a chance to move on in a healthy way.

Moving on in a healthy way means recovering *personally* from the affair so that you can pursue the future you want. It means knowing enough about what happened and *why* it happened to make a wise decision about whether to stay together or part. It means protecting yourself from being hurt again without carrying the backbreaking—and heartbreaking—burden of anger and suspicion or guilt and shame for the rest of your life.

The key is the adage "Everything in its time." In this book you'll find a chronological process that has helped hundreds of our clients move on from an affair in a healthy way. It's a methodical but flexible program, and we know it works, because it's based on the only treatment for infidelity that has been scientifically evaluated, a treatment that grew out of more than 50 years of our collective clinical experience and that we've taught to other therapists for the past decade. Besides being university professors and researchers, all three of us are clinical psychologists and therapists who specialize in working with couples having relationship difficulties, infidelity being one of our major areas of work. We've also written numerous articles and conducted frequent workshops for therapists in the United States and abroad on helping couples who are struggling to recover from an affair. All of this experience has gone into the program you'll read about here.

Why should you undertake this work, especially when you're feeling so beaten down by the trauma of the affair? **Because the issues you're wrestling with right now won't just go away with time**. If you simply try to wait out the pain, or tackle problems and issues in the wrong order, you can easily make decisions you'll regret. You can certainly end up with unresolved hurt and anger. Right after an affair is revealed, the most important tasks are to find a way to cope with the emotional turmoil and to know how to get through the day with your partner without making things worse or letting the rest of your life fall apart. Then, and only then, should you start to take a close look at your partner, yourself, and your history together so that you can figure out what made your relationship vulnerable to an affair and how you could change things in the future so that this marriage or a future one is on more solid ground. But this *is* work you should do, to whatever extent you feel able. Our experience has shown conclusively that this is the best way to emerge whole after an affair. Following the program in this book will leave you with a new understanding of yourself and your partner. You may emerge with a new view of what it means to be in a committed relationship and what the ideal partner looks like. And, though you may not believe it right now, if this turns out to be what you want, you very well could end up with a relationship that's stronger and better than it was before the affair.

Who Can Use This Book?

- This book is for anyone who has experienced an affair. Currently about 20% of men and 10% of women (and more women than ever before) engage in sexual infidelity at some point in their lives—and nearly 45% of men and 25% of women when emotional (nonsexual) affairs are included.

- An affair involves violating the expectations or standards of a relationship by becoming emotionally or physically involved with someone else, no matter what word you use to define it. You may think of this event in your life as an affair, infidelity, betrayal, outside involvement, tryst, one-night stand, or something else, depending on its duration or intensity and whether it was primarily sexual, primarily emotional, or—as is usually the case—both.

- You stand to gain from this book whether the affair was just revealed or you've been struggling with it for some time.

- The book will help you recover whether you're the injured partner (the one who did *not* have the affair) or the participating partner (the one who did). When we say "you," here and in the rest of this book, most of the time we mean the injured partner. Our work has shown that injured partners are *generally* more traumatized by an affair than participating partners, and therefore they're more likely to seek help. That's why we address you in particular through most of this book. But at times we'll also address the person who had the affair (and we'll make clear when we're doing so), as well as the two of you as a couple. We need to talk to your partner too because we know from our work that you stand the best chance of emerging whole and healthy when you both gain a full understanding of what happened.

- You can benefit from doing the work in this book whether you do it alone or with your partner. If your partner reads it too, even if the two of you work through it separately, *you* will be the beneficiary. Participants in affairs need to be honest with themselves about whether they're ready to end all involvement with the outside person. They need to figure out how to express care for their partners once the affair is over, as well as remorse. It's important that they understand why they ended up getting involved in an affair. If your partner explores these issues, trust and intimacy may grow between you again.

• This book is for you if you're in a committed relationship, whether you're married or not. We refer to marriage often because married couples are most likely to seek help.

How Should You Use This Book?

Ideally, both you and your partner will read each chapter and work through the program. You can do much of the suggested work separately, but some of it involves having conversations or engaging in activities together that will help you move forward. Still, we know that reality is rarely ideal, and you may end up working through this book alone for different reasons. Maybe your partner is one of those people who really don't like "self-help" books. Or perhaps your partner refuses to discuss what's happened. Or possibly you've already ended your relationship with your partner because of an affair, but you want to explore the experience on your own. That's a wise move, because there's plenty of research (including our own) that suggests that if traumatic relationship events such as an affair aren't addressed adequately, their negative impact could affect future relationships. If you have children with your partner, reading this book may help you resolve lingering resentments that might otherwise spill over into your co-parenting relationship and negatively affect your children.

Whether for these reasons or any others you plan to use this book on your own, your personal insights and increased understanding will put you in a better position to decide what to do about the future of your relationship if you're still with your partner. Moreover, once you learn to think about the affair and approach your life differently, you can change your relationship even if your partner isn't involved in making the same efforts. Although two people working together to make changes are often more effective than one, even one is better than none. So read this book for yourself and for your relationship—current or future. If you're involved in individual counseling while reading this book, share what you're reading with your counselor and together explore how this material applies to you.

We've presented the chapters in the order that has been most helpful to the couples we've counseled, and the chapters generally build on each other, but if certain questions seem particularly important to you, go ahead and read in whatever order you wish.

What Will You Gain?

From all the couples we've ushered through this process, we know that your first challenge is to deal with the initial devastation by avoiding further damage and managing essential tasks in the home.

Part I is about coping with the immediate trauma. It will help you:

- Deal with intense feelings—your own and your partner's.
- Communicate about extremely difficult topics.
- Decide how to go on with your daily routine, from managing chores and finances to parenting.
- Figure out how to keep living together while you regroup (should you sleep together? have sex?)—and under what limited circumstances an immediate separation makes sense.
- Establish boundaries with the outside affair person (i.e., the one with whom the participating partner had the affair)—who may not want to end the affair.
- Determine how much, if anything, to share with others about the affair—including your children, family members, or close friends.
- Take care of yourself even when it seems like your lowest priority, including getting help from friends and seeing your doctor when you need to.

Once you and your partner have restored some equilibrium to your relationship, Part II will help you examine all the factors that might have made your relationship vulnerable to an affair. It will help you:

- Look clearly at your relationship over the years—whether it's fulfilled your dreams, how it's changed, whether its foundations were shaken, and by what.
- Understand the characteristics and events that led one of you to have an affair.

- Understand what "infidelity" really means—and how boundaries can get crossed without any intention of hurting one's partner.
- Recognize how your environment, events, and other people helped set the stage.
- Understand how the injured partner can unwittingly contribute to a relationship's vulnerability—without being responsible for the participating partner's decision to have an affair.
- Avoid the temptation to be content with incomplete or partly accurate explanations just to avoid delving deeply into difficult topics.
- Arrive at a coherent picture or "narrative" of the affair that makes sense.

Part III guides you in making good decisions about moving forward—either separately or together. It will help you:

- Consider what it means to "move on" and how to get past disabling hurt feelings.
- Anticipate and deal with setbacks, whether together or apart.
- Continue strengthening your relationship and minimizing future risks if you've decided to stay together.

Although we don't presume to know what decisions you'll make down the road, we're confident that working through this book will lead you through a healthy process as you make the journey. We hope it will help ease the pain and uncertainty along the way. Right now, just understanding what's happened, figuring out how to get through the day, and hurting less are important goals. So let's get started.

Part I

HOW DO WE STOP HURTING?

What's Happening to Us?

"It's been three weeks since I found out. In some ways, it feels like it just happened, and at the same time it feels like this is going on forever. I've cried all the tears that I can cry, but then I find myself closing the door at work because I'm about to break down again. I lie in bed alone at night unable to sleep although I'm exhausted; in my mind I see my husband with her, and I think I'm going to throw up. I know I'm jumpy and irritable, and the kids must think I've turned into a monster. I can't concentrate, and I'm forgetting things at home and at work. We talk, we avoid each other—it doesn't matter. Nothing's working. One minute I want to kick him out of the house for what he's done; the next moment I want him to hold me and make it go away. I don't trust him about anything anymore—I even started checking his cell phone bills and his e-mails to see if he's contacting her again. This isn't the man I married. I've lost my sense of security; nothing fits together anymore."

What's Going On with Me?

If you've just learned that your partner has had an affair, you're struggling with one of the most traumatic experiences a person can face. (If you're the person who had the affair, you're also struggling, and we'll talk about that later in the chapter.) There are all kinds of traumatic events—from floods or plane crashes to infidelity. Any of these can be overwhelming.

But natural disasters and mechanical failure are unintentional and typically unavoidable. A partner's affair results from deliberate decisions by your *partner*—the one person who's supposed to love and care for you, protect you from the rest of the world, and treat you with respect, dignity, and honesty. For many people, few betrayals can be more hurtful and disruptive.

Understanding the impact of traumatic events and how most people recover from them can help you develop a larger picture of what's happening to you and your partner and what's likely to happen to you both in the future. So, first, what *is* a traumatic event?

>>> **A trauma is a major negative event or set of events that destroys important assumptions or fundamental beliefs about the world or specific people—in this case, your partner and your relationship.**
Traumatic events disrupt all parts of your life—your thoughts, feelings, and behaviors.

You assumed that your relationship would be safe and that your well-being would be uppermost in your partner's mind, both when you were together and when you were apart. You trusted that your partner valued you and your relationship. You expected honesty—that no large parts of your partner's life would be hidden from you. Finally, you expected your partner to honor commitments you made to each other—whether stated out loud or just understood. Most likely one of those commitments involved reserving certain behaviors for the two of you—specifically, sexual or intimate behavior and sharing of certain information or feelings. When those commitments are violated, we feel violated ourselves.

Why does the dashing of those assumptions hit us so hard? Because we all rely on certain assumptions to get through the day with minimal effort. When your partner tells you something, you don't want to have to stop and evaluate whether it's the truth. If your partner comes home late, you don't want to wonder whether the meeting really ran late or have to check up on where he or she was. And if you think your partner was unfair about something, you want the freedom to get upset or express your anger without having to worry that you'll be left for someone else. Your assumptions about your partner and your relationship make your life together safe and predictable. When they're shattered, you're thrown off balance, disoriented and unsure of how to get your bearings.

The effects of this trauma take a variety of forms, some of them surprising, in your thoughts, feelings, and behavior. Can you identify with any of the common reactions listed in the box on page 12? We'll go into more detail on them in the following pages, because understanding these reactions is critical. (Exercise 1.1 at the end of this chapter can assist you in this.) Your partner's affair doesn't just violate the mutual commitment to reserving sex and romantic love for each other. It calls into question every other assumption about your partner and your relationship: "If you lied about this, what else are you lying about? If you're going to do what you want without regard for me even in this most intimate part of our life, are you just going to do whatever you want in other areas too?"

When important assumptions are violated in one aspect of your relationship, the whole relationship can be thrown out of balance. That's why you might feel the way so many people struggling with a partner's affair feel:

"I feel like the rug has been pulled out from under me. I don't believe anything anymore."

"I've lost my bearings. I'm totally confused and disoriented."

"I don't know my partner anymore. This just isn't the person I thought I married. How could this happen?"

You may start questioning your assumptions about yourself as well:

"How could I be such a fool? I can't trust my own judgment anymore."

"How could I miss seeing it? I think some of my friends were trying to warn me, but I just wouldn't listen."

"Did I fall short as a partner? Did I get so busy and distracted that I didn't see what I was doing? What was wrong with *me*?"

Research indicates that people are at high risk for developing significant depression and anxiety after experiencing a betrayal such as an affair, just as they would after any significant loss. Affairs bring about many losses—loss of safety and predictability, loss of dreams for your relationship and perhaps for your future, loss of innocence, loss of trust. These are on top of the loss of something special and unique that you two shared exclusively: sex, romance, and your innermost thoughts and feelings.

Common Reactions to Learning about a Partner's Affair

Common Thoughts

- You question previous beliefs about your partner—for example, no longer viewing your partner as caring or trustworthy.
- Your beliefs about the relationship are shattered—for example, you no longer view your relationship as a source of support or fulfillment.
- You adopt extreme, negative explanations for your partner's behavior—for example, thinking your partner *wanted* to hurt you deeply.
- You have doubts about your future with your partner.
- You harbor fears that other betrayals may remain hidden or lie ahead.
- You have the sense that your relationship is beyond your control—that you have little influence over what happens between you and your partner.

Common Feelings

- You feel strong, overwhelming emotions such as anger, depression, and anxiety.
- You feel foolish, ashamed, or guilty.
- You're uncertain about your own worth or attractiveness.
- You feel profoundly vulnerable and unsafe.
- Your feelings are unpredictable, possibly changing daily or hourly.
- You experience flashbacks in which you reexperience painful feelings, memories, or images from the affair (discussed further in Chapter 2).
- You're confused about what you feel and about what you want either now or in the future.
- You feel as though your emotions can overwhelm you or are out of your control.
- You have periods of numbness when you don't feel much of anything at all.

Common Behaviors

- You act disoriented—for example, staring off or wandering about for extended periods with no apparent purpose or direction.
- You retreat emotionally or physically—for example, withdrawing into prolonged silence or avoiding interaction and seeking separate space.
- You persistently seek an explanation of your partner's behavior—for example, repeatedly asking, "How could you do this?"
- You seek revenge—for example, attacking your partner verbally or physically, destroying your partner's property, or harming his or her relationships with others.
- You try to reassure yourself—for example, initiating frequent and intense sexual encounters with your partner in an attempt to make up for your partner's previous complaints about your sexual relationship.

You might experience a wide range of other negative feelings as well, from anger to anxiety and fear or even guilt. Anger is a common reaction to believing you've been treated unfairly, and affairs feel extremely unfair. Your partner chose to cheat, lie, cover up, and perhaps put you at risk for a sexually transmitted disease. Does your anger make sense? Absolutely. Fear and anxiety arise when your world feels unsafe and unpredictable. A partner's affair breaks down all the protective walls, and suddenly nothing feels safe or predictable anymore. Guilt usually results when you think you're to blame or have done something wrong. In trying to make sense of a partner's affair, some people conclude, "It must be me. At some level, it must be my fault." Those feelings, too, are understandable, but make no mistake about it: *Your partner's affair isn't your fault.* In Part II of this book we'll help you explore your own role in creating your relationship with your partner. But people have to take responsibility for their own individual behavior—and that certainly includes your partner's decision to have an affair.

On a fundamental level, an affair throws your normal emotional state into total disarray. Your feelings might change from one minute to the next. Or they might be so jumbled together that you don't know what you feel. Maybe you're not really feeling much of anything—and think there must be something wrong with you because you're not. Research suggests that a trauma is often followed by an initial sense of numbness, possibly as a way of protecting ourselves from being overwhelmed by intense feelings. In most cases, those feelings surface at some later point. Or you might be someone who doesn't experience emotions strongly; people react differently to traumatic events.

If you're one of those people who *is* experiencing a lot of strong emotion, your behavior is likely to be out of character or at times even chaotic. When you can no longer trust or believe what you've always taken as a given, you're not likely to act the way you used to either. You might find yourself shouting at a grocery store clerk for no good reason or showing up unannounced at your partner's office to talk—only to change your mind and leave abruptly. Or you may find yourself driving toward the outside affair person's house or place of business, not entirely clear about what you would do or say if you were to confront that person. Research suggests that an individual may even become physically aggressive toward his or her partner or the outside person during this time. Todd felt as though he'd lost all self-control after discovering Mika's affair three weeks ago. He found himself yelling at coworkers in meetings over trivial issues; at home he was short-tempered with his children. Even worse was the shameful memory of punching Mika's lover during a confrontation outside a local coffee shop. While anger is common, such aggression is obviously problematic and can potentially be dangerous. If you're struggling with managing your anger, you may want to jump ahead to the guidelines for handling strong emotions in Chapter 3.

Your usual daily routines developed within a relationship that had predictability and meaning. Now that relationship has been called into question. Are you really going to get up and make coffee for someone who betrayed you? You used to give each other a peck on the cheek when you left in the morning—nothing passionate, just a sign that you loved each other and were partners. A simple peck on the cheek is no longer simple. Now if your partner touches you, you may cringe as it brings back painful memories, or you might want to sink into an embrace, trying to feel connected again. Should you still go out to dinner together with friends? If so, are you cold and distant, or do you pretend to be the happy couple while inside you want to die? Behaviors you took for granted, which had become routine and almost automatic, now seem awkward, disgusting, or unsafe.

The bottom line is that a partner's affair is a big deal. *It's traumatic.* It involves violations of core assumptions about your partner, your relationship, and perhaps even yourself. You can anticipate a wide variety of feelings, most of them negative. And at times you're going to say and do things that just aren't like you. It's miserable. It feels awful. But it's also a normal reaction to what's happened. And our research and clinical work with couples strongly suggest that if you go through the recovery process in a healthy manner, these feelings won't remain as strong as they are right now, and they won't be there all the time. Things can get better.

What's Happening to Us?

Part of what's happening to you as a couple right now is a direct result of the turmoil that's going on with each of you individually. Let's face it: No matter how well your partner might be managing his or her own feelings, your relationship isn't likely to go well when you're still struggling with the initial trauma of finding out about the affair. You're not likely to express yourself effectively. You're probably not able to listen in a caring way to your partner's views. You may find it difficult to collaborate on even routine tasks such as paying bills together, making decisions about the children, dealing with a car that needs repair, or the hundreds of other mundane chores involved in having a committed partnership. And when these tasks get put aside, the negative consequences of neglecting them can bring additional stress. The phone company threatens to disconnect your phone; one of the kids gets into trouble at school; the rattle under the hood turns into a major engine overhaul, with no money to pay for it.

All that can happen even when your partner is handling his own feelings reasonably well. Chances are he isn't. Independent of what you're feeling, your partner is probably struggling with his own turmoil. Right now, you may have too much of your own hurt or anger to be very sympathetic. That's understandable. But at some point, if you want to be able to interact more effectively, you're going to need a better understanding of what your partner is experiencing. Reading the material on pages 20–24, where we speak to your partner, might be helpful when you decide you want to gain more of this understanding. But for now, just consider that your partner is probably wrestling with difficult feelings too—possibly including confusion and uncertainty about the future, anxiety about your relationship, aloneness, hurt, anger, guilt, or shame. In fact, even if *you* are managing your own feelings well, there's a good chance your relationship would still be feeling crazy because of what's going on with your partner right now.

Mix together these two factors—your own turmoil and your partner's—and you have the perfect formula for chaos. Just when you feel able to talk constructively, your partner won't. And just when your partner feels able to approach you or respond constructively, you can't. Moreover, whatever feelings either one of you is struggling with at any given moment can trigger equally intense and difficult feelings in the other.

To understand why this happens, it's helpful to think of your interactions as serving three functions—communication, protection, and restoration—each of which is thwarted by the trauma of the affair:

1. It's too hard for your partner to hear what you feel has to be said. You want your partner to understand the trauma caused by the affair. Those feelings are intense, sometimes exceeding your ability to express them. And if your partner cares for you at all, hearing you express these feelings will be uncomfortable or even painful. After all, it's your partner who is the source of the trauma. So your partner may eventually pull back or stop listening as intently when you continue to express your feelings.

At that point you're likely to feel unheard, and you're going to crank up the volume. But a person who already feels on the defensive or overwhelmed by the intensity of your feelings is going to pull back even further, and you're going to feel even less heard and less understood. It's a vicious cycle of wanting to be understood and, instead, feeling less and less heard by your partner.

2. The need to feel safe often means trying to protect yourselves from each other. In addition to wanting to be understood, both you and your partner want to feel safe. But you can't feel safe when you're afraid you might be hurt again. You've probably heard of the "fight or flight" response to threat. When you choose to "fight" in response to danger, you arm yourself, go on the offensive, and keep others away by threatening to do them harm. So, in an effort to protect yourself you may sometimes punish your partner such as through verbal attacks: "How could you be so cruel? I hate you." "Where was your integrity? Just wait until I tell the children." Aggressively pursuing control can be another way to "fight" your way to safety: "You're never going anywhere again without my knowing where and without your checking in." "You can't be trusted; I want our bank accounts signed over to me." Physical aggression can be still another way of seeking safety, even when initiated by someone who's physically smaller and less powerful. It's a way of saying, "Stay away from me unless you want to get hurt." Unfortunately, fighting isn't very effective at restoring a damaged relationship. It's not even a great way to ensure safety. Attacks can lead to counterattacks.

Some safety-seeking partners opt for "flight" instead of "fight," retreating physically by demanding separate bedrooms or separate living quarters or retreating verbally—withdrawing into silence and refusing to interact. Other kinds of retreat can be more subtle. Faye desperately wanted to forgive Joe's affair and made every effort to put it behind her. But her feelings of insecurity and anger continued to gnaw at her, and she found herself avoiding being alone with Joe. Joe noticed her retreat and complained about their lack of intimacy, but Faye didn't know what to do about it. Some couples end up leading a civil life together but really talk only about superficial things, ignoring more difficult relationship issues.

What can make this all very complicated and confusing is that your efforts to create safety can run afoul of each other. For example, when your questioning triggers an angry defense from your partner, each of you is trying to feel safer but instead ends up feeling more threatened. Or there may be times when you've pulled back into silence and your partner tries to reassure you, but the approach feels too scary for you and you use anger to push your partner away.

3. It's not just the thought that counts in efforts to restore the relationship—it's applying the right strategies at the right time. Each of you may be trying in your own way to restore your relationship, but these efforts just aren't working. Those who have participated in an affair often try to restore the marriage by convincing the injured partner that the affair didn't really mean anything or that they're totally committed to the relationship but just didn't realize it before. Injured partners sometimes try to restore their relationship by cutting off the affair outsider, by trying to push thoughts of the affair completely out of their minds, or by finding out "why" the partner had the affair. Such attempts may ultimately reflect the right goal, but they can fall short unless they are well thought through:

- **Is this the right move?** Sometimes efforts backfire, doing more damage instead of restoring the relationship. For example, trying to promote closeness by insisting that you and your partner do everything together may instead make your partner feel suffocated and desperate to escape.
- **Is it the right time?** Even fundamentally good strategies have to be implemented in the right order. Insistence on exploring factors that led to the affair, while ultimately a crucial part of restoring long-term security to your relationship, won't be constructive if one of you still feels deeply misunderstood or emotionally vulnerable to the other.

Fortunately, both ineffective strategies and poor timing often can be avoided. In fact, the whole purpose of this book is to provide you with effective strategies for communicating, reestablishing safety, and restoring individual and relationship security—and implementing these strategies in a sequence and time frame that are more likely to be successful.

Do We Have a Future Together?

This question may be the most important issue you're facing right now. Can you and your partner truly recover? Can you restore a trusting, loving relationship and move on together to bring each other joy and enrich one another's life?

Our answer to this is "Maybe." We can tell you that among married couples in which one member has recently learned of the partner's affair, only a minority go on to divorce. Most, approximately 60–75%, remain married. Among couples who stay together, many go on to restore a loving and secure relationship. But some couples struggling to recover from an affair remain married yet continue feeling hurt, distrustful, and very unhappy.

At this point you're undoubtedly struggling with so many confusing emotions that you don't even know whether you both *want* to stay together. That's fine. Just keep in mind that eventually you'll have to figure out what you both want in addition to what's possible. As to what determines who restores a secure relationship and who doesn't, we emphasized in the Introduction that **couples need to accomplish three critical tasks:**

1. Find ways to manage and minimize the painful emotions.
2. Come to understand how the affair came about.
3. Reach an explicit, informed decision about how to move forward.

Right now you and your partner need to concentrate on task number one, finding ways of surviving the immediate crisis, because it's difficult to start exploring what happened when you're preoccupied by confusing and troubling emotions and don't know how to interact with your partner anymore. This requires managing strong feelings to address a lot of practical decisions in addition to simply taking better care of yourself: Should you touch each other, sleep together, make love? How do you handle anger? How do you start talking about the affair without making things worse? What do you do when your daily routine is disrupted by repeated memories or "flashbacks" of the affair? How do you deal with the outside affair person, and what will you tell your children and others, if anything?

Once you've addressed these issues, you've cleared a path for determining what happened that led you to this situation. What placed your relationship at risk for an affair? What has to happen so you can eliminate or reduce those risks in the future? How can you assure yourselves and each other of your commitment to pursuing these changes? **Answering these questions is difficult, without a doubt, but lies at the**

very heart of recovery. You'll have to be willing to look closely at your relationship, at things that were happening outside your relationship, at your partner and even yourself if you're to get complete answers. As we said earlier, you're *not* responsible for your partner's infidelity, but it's important to find out whether you contributed to an environment ripe for an affair.

> *For example, determined but sometimes painful exploration led Liz to conclude that there were some early warning signs of Jerry's emotional withdrawal before he had an affair with the wife of a family friend, but at the time these felt too threatening to Liz to confront directly. To eliminate the danger of the same sequence unfolding in the future, Liz ultimately agreed that she would ask Jerry if her fears were accurate if she saw the same signs again, and Jerry agreed that he would address her concerns directly and honestly. Both agreed to work at expressing and responding to such concerns without anger. Each pledged to protect their relationship from situations that had placed them at risk for an affair in the past, and they committed to making their marriage their top priority. But it took time and effort to get to this point. The reward, both felt, was worth it all: They reestablished the emotional security that's critical to an intimate relationship.*

With that emotional security in place, Liz and Jerry were able to reconcile, as many other couples are too. But the goal of doing this work is to reach a healthy, informed decision about how to move on, and that doesn't necessarily mean reconciliation. People can work through this recovery process by restoring their relationship to its previous form, by changing and strengthening it, or by ending it. By "moving on" we mean that each of you will be able to move beyond focusing almost exclusively on the affair and will voluntarily stop punishing each other. Instead, you'll each be able to redirect your efforts toward an emotionally satisfying and productive life. This affair will never be forgotten. But it will no longer dominate your lives.

The step-by-step process for recovering from an affair we outline in this book has helped hundreds of couples move forward in a healthier way. Most—about 70%—choose to rebuild their relationship. Many of these— nearly half—restore an intimate relationship that's stronger than it was before the affair. Other couples find this process helpful but may continue to struggle with individual or relationship problems that were present long before the affair—such as sexual dysfunctions, substance use, deep depression, or other emotional or behavioral difficulties. Some individuals working through the process outlined here decide to end their relationship and move on separately. Among these, many discover that their improved understanding of themselves and others allows them to develop a stronger, deeper relationship with a new partner.

Whether you move on together or separately is something we encourage you to decide later, after you've finished obtaining a more complete understanding of what's happened. If you and your partner have already reached a long-term decision about your relationship, that's okay. But we'd still suggest that you hold the decision "open" and revisit it from time to time as you gain new information and understanding.

In reaching any decision, it's important to understand what was happening with both of you that set the stage for an affair. If you feel ready to consider some of what your partner might be experiencing in all of this at present, read on. If you don't feel receptive to that right now, put the book away for a while and come back to it when you're ready. Ultimately, to move on with your own recovery process, you'll want to continue from here and understand your partner better. It's not uncommon that our most intimate and rewarding relationships are also the source of our deepest hurt and disappointment. However, recovery from even the most profound relationship heartaches *can* occur. The process we've outlined in this book will help.

For the Participating Partner

"I know I've screwed up; that's not the problem. The problem is, I don't know how to make it right again. I'm doing everything I know how to get us back on track. But nothing seems to work. She wants to talk about the affair, and I don't. Talking about it just seems to get her more upset. But if I don't talk about it, she thinks I'm trying to hide something, or that I don't understand how hurt she is, or I just don't care enough to work on it. Sure I care. That's why I'm trying to avoid these awful arguments we get into every time she asks questions about how I cheated on her. We go over and over the same old stuff. I don't know if there's anything I can do at this point to make things better."

How Can I Be Helpful?

If your partner has recently learned about your affair, and you're reading this book, you've already taken a critical step toward being helpful.

>>> **The most important things you can communicate to your partner right now are that:**
   - **You want to understand what's happening to each of you.**
   - **You're willing to take a hard look at how this affair came about.**
   - **You want to figure out the best way to move on.**

That's what this book is all about. It's going to take patience, commitment to the entire process, and lots of hard work. But continuing to read through the next few pages is an important first step.

You may not be willing to do this. Some people who've had an affair already have their bags packed and have one foot out the door. Others apologize and take their punishment but don't really want to do any additional work to make the relationship right again. And even if you *are* willing, you and your partner might not be able to make your relationship survive despite patience, commitment, and hard work. Affairs happen for all kinds of reasons, to all kinds of people in all kinds of circumstances. So we couldn't begin to tell you at this point whether your relationship can—or should—be saved.

As mentioned above, some couples stay together; some don't. Of the couples that stay together, some go on to build a better and stronger relationship; others stay together but remain hurt, angry, distrustful, and generally miserable. The same is true for couples who break up or divorce following an affair. For partners who've done the work to know themselves better, understand their own needs and vulnerabilities, and find a way of placing their own or their partner's affair into a bigger life-picture, moving on separately can sometimes permit new, healthier relationships to develop. But for partners who divorce out of anger, confusion, or just not knowing a process for making good decisions, life after a divorce can continue to feel as hurtful or as empty as the relationship did following the affair.

How can you help the recovery process? For now, we invite you to take three very important steps. None may be easy. Each might be more difficult than the one listed just before it.

1. Work at understanding your partner's experience. If you haven't done so already, go back and read this chapter from the beginning. You're going to read about how your affair has impacted your partner. Reading this might be uncomfortable or even painful. But an important message you'll be communicating to your partner is this: "I want to understand how you're feeling right now. Sometimes it's hard for me to listen to you when you're so angry, or to ask about your feelings when you've pulled back into silence. But I do want to understand so I'll know better how to respond."

2. Commit to a recovery *process*. You and your partner don't need to decide right now whether to stay in this relationship for the long term. Instead, we encourage you to commit the necessary time and effort to understand the impact of your affair, explore the various reasons for it, and then decide with your partner how you can each move on to a full and enriching life—together or separately.

3. Avoid doing more damage. As obvious as this step sounds, it can be the most difficult of all. Right now, both you and your partner might have some very strong feelings. It's easy to escalate into heated arguments. It's easy to be misunderstood. It's hard to avoid falling into the trap of attacks and counterattacks. In the next three chapters, we're going to give you some concrete steps for avoiding doing more damage. But for now, specific things to do are:

- *Be patient.* If you expect recovery to be quick, you're going to be frustrated. If you expect your partner to get over it, you're going to be disappointed. And if you require yourself to be perfect in your own responses, you're going to feel disillusioned.
- *Be truthful.* Continued dishonesty, deception, and half-truths ultimately will be more destructive than your affair itself. This doesn't mean that you have to disclose every detail of your affair; that can also be destructive. But if you say something, be sure it's the truth. If your partner asks you a question and you're not yet willing to answer, just say so: "I know this is important to you. And I don't want any more secrets or dishonesty. But I'm not able to talk with you about this yet."
- *Be trusting.* Specifically, trust the process. We're confident that if each of you commits to the process we're going to take you through in this book, you're each going to end up in a better

place—less hurt, less angry, and better equipped to move on and lead a happier life again.

What about Me?

Marcus had been feeling hurt and neglected by Lucia, who seemed to be completely wrapped up in their new baby and too tired to even think about sex. He thought visiting a sexually explicit chat room on the Internet would be a safe outlet and never expected to arrange to meet someone in person. It just felt so good to be wanted, and a small part of him felt angry and justified in his behavior. Later, when he looked back on the experience, he felt dirty and ashamed. How could he do that to his new family? What had come over him?

Your partner's probably not the only one who feels misunderstood. There's a good chance you do too. You might be feeling one or more of the following:

- *Confused.* "How did I get into this mess? How do I get out of it? How do I make things right again?"
- *Hurt.* "Can't she see that I didn't intend to hurt her? What more can I say? Why can't she accept my apology?"
- *Angry.* "It's not all me. Yes, I'm the one who had the affair. But this relationship was far from perfect, and he had a lot to do with that. I'm tired of taking all the blame and punishment for this mess. Enough is enough."
- *Guilty or ashamed.* "I deserve whatever I get. I want her to forgive me and move on, but that's probably too much to hope for and certainly too much to ask. I can't stand to hear her talk about her feelings about the affair; it makes me feel terrible, like I'm a heartless jerk or something. I wish she'd just let it be."
- *Alone.* "If I thought I was alone before, that was nothing compared to how I feel now. Right now I have no one. I don't know how much longer I can go on this way."
- *Uncertain.* "I just don't know for sure what I want. I know having an affair wasn't the right answer to whatever problems or feelings I was having before. But I'm not sure what the right answer is or how to find it."

During the process you're about to undertake, you'll be addressing difficult feelings and questions that you and your partner both have—whether you're working together as a couple or separately by yourself. Early in this process, your partner might have difficulty listening to what you need or how you feel. Your partner might feel that your relationship is already unbalanced and you've been focusing mostly on what *you* want. As you move through this process and are able to listen to your partner's hurt and pain, often your partner can start to do the same in hearing from you.

So we encourage you to be patient and truthful and to trust in the process. We're not going to ask you and your partner to do this all at once. We're going to take you through the process step-by-step. However, as therapists we've experienced the remarkable strengths that both partners can bring to a damaged relationship when they're given a process for doing so. ***We've worked with many couples whose marriages actually ended up stronger, more faithful, and more personally fulfilling for both spouses after the affair.*** We hope that this will also be true for the two of you.

What's Next?

Whether you're the injured or the participating partner, do the exercises on the following pages. If you're reading this book alone and want your partner's involvement, we encourage you to approach your partner and say something like the following: "I know this is really difficult, but I want us to find a way of working through this situation. I found a book that I think could help us. I've read the first chapter, and much of it makes sense to me. Please read through the first chapter and let me know when you're finished. I need to know whether we can commit to a process that can help us work together to move forward." Find a way to express your wish as an invitation or request, not as a threat or demand. What's important is that the message comes out of your sincere concern for your partner and your relationship. Neither of you needs to commit to anything other than the wish that you'll each be able to recover and move on toward a fruitful and happy life.

If your partner still won't join you in working through the recovery process outlined in this book, there are three important things you can still do:

1. *Work through this book on your own.* Begin by working through this first set of exercises to reach for your own personal recovery. You could end up restoring this relationship through your own understanding of what's happened and how to prevent it from happening again. Or, if you end this relationship, your own recovery will leave you better able to pursue a satisfying life single or as part of a new couple.

2. *Don't give up hope.* Your own personal recovery can demonstrate the positive effects of the process and demonstrate to your partner the benefits of joining you in it. Both the research and our clinical experience have shown that in at least half of the cases in which the injured partner started out working alone toward recovery, hope for the relationship was renewed and the partner who had the affair made new efforts to participate.

3. *Do the end-of-chapter exercises by yourself.* Some are designed for you as an individual; others will be for you as a couple. In many cases you can do the couple exercises if you just change them a bit; we'll help you do that.

Exercises

The goal of the exercises at the end of each chapter is to help you take what you've been reading and apply it to your own situation. You'll move closer toward recovery as you bring these ideas to life in your own relationship.

Some exercises will suggest that you write things down. We recommend that you create a notebook where you keep your responses, no matter how brief or how detailed. If you're working with your partner, it might be good for each of you to have a separate notebook. For the exercise that follows for this chapter, we recommend that even if you and your partner are working through the book together, you do it separately and not share your responses with each other for now. Take some time by yourself to look at what's happening for you right now.

At times later in the book, we'll suggest you go back and see how things have changed during this journey, so writing down your responses can help you see your progress. Take whatever time you need for each exercise. Give yourself the gift of time to focus and understand, and to plan for the future.

EXERCISE 1.1.
UNDERSTANDING YOUR REACTIONS TO WHAT'S HAPPENED

Before you can change something, you need to be aware of what's happening. For now, we want to make sure you know what's happening to you individually. Later we'll ask you to try to understand your partner and the affair.

Feelings

What are the main feelings you're having now and since the affair was discovered or disclosed? Are you angry, sad, or frightened? Confused or numb? Relieved at having it in the open? Have you had any good feelings as you've talked with your partner—warm, close, reassured, or some other feelings?

List your major feelings and try to link them to what you're thinking at the time or to what's just happened. For example:

> "I get furious when he refuses to talk to me about what happened. He owes me that much."

> "I get really frightened and anxious when I think about what may lie ahead. Will I have my relationship? Have I blown it for good?"

> "I get frustrated when he asks me the same questions night after night; is he just trying to punish me?"

> "As we've talked, we've both realized how precious and how fragile life and relationships are. It's made us realize how much we want to make this work; it's crazy, but with all the pain, at times I feel closer than I did before."

Thoughts and Assumptions

Affairs not only make you feel bad; they also tear away some of your core beliefs about your partner, your relationship, and maybe even yourself. We want you to see clearly what upsets you most about what's happened.

List your major beliefs or views about your partner, your relationship, or yourself that have been questioned or destroyed as a result of the affair. For example:

"What's most upsetting to me is that I thought he was the one person in my life I could count on to care for me; now I know I can't."

"When we got married, we said we'd always be totally honest with each other. I've done that; she hasn't. I can never trust her again."

"If anyone had asked me before this happened what I thought about infidelity, I'd have said it's wrong and will never happen to us. Now, I've done this horrible thing. I've always considered myself a good and honorable person. I guess I was wrong."

You also might have had some new and positive thoughts since this happened; please list those as well. For example:

"I always thought I was weak and couldn't make it on my own. Since I've had to face that possibility, I've realized I can make it through almost anything. I'm actually much stronger than I realized."

Behaviors

When you and your partner are this upset, you might behave uncharacteristically. This is understandable, given the situation, but if you continue behaving this way for long, things probably won't get better or will get worse.

List the major ways that you've started behaving differently as an individual that might get in the way of recovery or are making things worse. For example:

"I've started yelling, calling her horrible names, and attacking her. I've never been this way. Not only do I not like her right now, I don't like how I'm behaving either."

"I'm withdrawing even though I know we have to talk. But I don't know if I can have those conversations; it's just too painful."

You might also be acting in some new ways that you feel good about. List those too. For example:

"It's always been hard for me to stand up for myself in our relationship. Somehow this affair has changed things. I'm standing up for myself now, and it feels good. Whether I stay in this relationship or not, I'll never allow anyone to mistreat me or ignore my needs again."

"I've always covered things up and never been totally honest. I'm doing it differently now. I'm being honest. If our relationship can't handle the honesty, then maybe it shouldn't last. In any case, although I'm ashamed of what I've done, I like the new, honest part of me."

2

How Do We
Get Through the Day?

Paula first suspected David's affair when a friend said she'd seen him having "an intimate dinner" with another woman when Paula was out of town. David seemed flustered when asked about it but insisted she was a business consultant from out of town he had been asked to entertain. When Paula learned a week later that this "consultant" lived in their own community, she was furious. David had confessed to a "one-night stand" several years earlier on a trip with his old high school buddies. But the couple had put it behind them and never really discussed it after the first couple of weeks. This time, Paula insisted that David move out.

At first, David and Paula continued to see each other after work to try to sort through what had happened. Paula insisted on knowing every detail of the affair, and initially David answered most of her questions. But when she demanded to know the other woman's name and address, David refused. For the next three weeks he stayed away and wouldn't return Paula's phone calls. When they finally talked again, Paula asked him to move back home so they could work things out. Moreover, the kids missed him and were starting to have problems at school. David agreed to do whatever he could to work on their relationship, but only on the condition that they wouldn't discuss his affair anymore.

Having a break from the heated arguments that arose whenever they discussed David's affair was a relief. But soon Paula still found herself wondering about the affair and questioning David's honesty. His kisses felt awkward; sex just didn't interest her. Quickly she ran out of excuses to avoid lovemaking, and David accused her of not really wanting to get close again. When he gave up on approaching her sexually, Paula only worried more about his commitment to their relationship. Before they knew it, they were hardly speaking. Neither one wanted a divorce, but it felt as if the gap between them was widening every day.

Right after an affair comes to light, life feels unsafe. Most couples describe their relationship as chaotic. Now that all the "givens" have been destroyed and the rules violated, they have no idea how to interact just to get through the day. How should you and your partner try to deal with what's happening in your relationship? How do you communicate without letting your feelings get out of control? What should you talk about? How do you manage routine activities like preparing meals, taking care of the children, or paying bills? How affectionate does either of you feel toward the other, and what should you do if you differ in this area? Most important, how do you and your partner avoid making things worse?

Couples usually react in one of three ways, and often they try various approaches because nothing seems to work:

1. Some couples try to go on as if nothing has happened and immediately attempt to put the affair behind them.
2. Other couples are frightened by the possibility that their relationship might end and increase their efforts to get close. They spend more time together, make love more often, and try to create in their relationship whatever closeness or passion might have been missing.
3. Still other couples feel they need to get away from each other, avoid each other, retreat to different corners of the house, or perhaps live apart for a while until the anger simmers down. Sometimes a separation can be a last resort for reducing endless arguments or is important in stopping physical aggression that destroys whatever chances the relationship had. But at other times a separation at this point can deepen mistrust, drive partners fur-

ther apart, and increase the outside person's access to the participating partner who may actually be trying to end the affair.

Here's the advice we often give couples trying to deal with the immediate aftermath of an affair: "For now, let's just focus on trying not to make
things worse. There's not a lot of *recovery* that's likely to happen right
now. But the chances of your recovering down the road could be strongly
affected by decisions you make about how to deal with things over the
next month or two." **Not making things worse is what this chapter and
the next two are all about.**

**Setting good boundaries is probably the most important way to
avoid making things worse.** You're going to need boundaries between
your partner and you, between you two and the outside affair person, and
between you two and other people who may or may not need to be told
about the affair. The boundaries you'll need first, just to get through each
day, are the ones between you and your partner, so these are discussed
here. But if you find that too many conversations quickly reach a boiling
point, that you can't seem to make the simplest decisions together, or that
you can't establish a constructive give-and-take between talking and listening when you try to share difficult feelings, turn to Chapter 3 for specific communication skills and strategies. And if the participating partner
is still struggling to end the affair—either because of ongoing strong feelings for the outsider or because the outside person doesn't want to let go,
or both—you may want to skip ahead and read the relevant portion of
Chapter 4 before reading the rest of this chapter.

Setting Boundaries between You and Your Partner

*"We just can't get away from it," Pam complained. "It's the same
thing every night. Question after question after question. Tom never
lets up. He's never satisfied with my answers, no matter what I say.
He always wants to know more. It feels like an inquisition. I can't take
it anymore. I know what I did was wrong. I've sworn to Tom and myself not to lie anymore. But some of the details feel so painful—not
just to me, but to Tom too. Our talks aren't making things better;
they're making things worse. But if I say, 'Enough!' and want to stop
for the night, he gets furious."*

Should We Talk about the Affair?

Most couples find it impossible *not* to talk about the affair. That would feel like being in the middle of a hurricane and not talking about how the roof is being torn away. Talking about the affair is one way of communicating hurt: "How could you do this?" Talking about the affair is a way of trying to reestablish security: "Have you lost your feelings for me? Isn't our marriage important to you anymore?" The trouble is, you and your partner may not agree about whether to talk about it or how much to discuss or reveal. It's important to understand what you do need to talk about and how to set boundaries that permit such discussions without allowing one partner to go so much farther that it can only make things worse. Exercise 2.1 at the end of this chapter will help you do this.

As difficult as it can be for people like Pam, talking about the affair is probably the only way of coming to a complete understanding of how the affair came about and what the chances are that it will happen again in the future. And not all couples do talk about a partner's affair—at least not initially. It's understandable why some couples try this approach. Talking about an affair is more than painful. It can be frightening as well: "The more I tell my partner about the affair, the more she'll realize just how deceptive and dishonest I was to keep it a secret." Or, "If I push too hard and force my partner to talk about her affair when she really doesn't want to, I may end up pushing her right out the door—and I'm really not ready for that." Sometimes a person is reluctant to discuss his or her affair because the partner's pain becomes even more evident at those times. It can be particularly painful when one person wants to discuss the affair and the other one doesn't. Fear of pain and fear of the unknown can be powerful barriers to discussing an affair, even if not facing these in the short run can ensure more difficulties in the long run.

When Pam confessed her affair to Tom, he said he was hurt but would try to understand. He asked that they both put the affair out of their minds and try to avoid thinking about it again. But then, months later, his attitude seemed to change. He wanted to know everything. How did Pam's lover kiss? What did they talk about when in bed together? Exactly what did they do sexually? The more vivid the images became, the more haunting they were. Soon he could think of nothing else. Pam and Tom struggled to distinguish between discussions they needed to have to reestablish emotional security and discussions they needed to avoid because they would likely make recovery more difficult.

What Do We Talk About and Not Talk About?

When a couple first begins to talk about one partner's affair, three overriding questions are important to consider:

- What happened?
- Why did you do it?
- Where does this leave us?

What Happened?

In discussing "what happened," couples need to reach a common understanding about the basic events of the affair. In the box on page 34 we've listed some common questions that couples usually need to address after a partner's infidelity. You need to know when the affair began, how long it lasted, and when and how it ended. For example, a one-time sexual encounter in unusual circumstances may have a different meaning and different effects on a relationship than a six-month affair with a close friend of the couple. Pam's affair was a weeklong "fling" that included one instance of sexual intimacy during Tom's two-month business trip in Europe. Although it was Pam's guilt that made her disclose her infidelity to her husband, in her mind it *could* be put behind them because it was such a fleeting event in their lives. Tom seemed to agree at first, but the emotional fallout turned out to be just as devastating as if it had gone on for months. The intensity and duration of an affair are important to get out in the open because these factors could have significant implications for the couple's moving forward.

You may also want and need to know something about the outside affair person and the nature of the affair in order to move forward. What was the outside person's role in initiating or maintaining the affair? Was the affair mostly emotional or sexual? Some research suggests that women sometimes find emotional involvement of their partners with someone else particularly threatening, whereas men often react more strongly to their partners' sexual involvement with someone else.

It's only natural to want to understand the "magnitude of threat" from an outside person, and that's why if you're the injured party you probably can't help focusing on what your partner and the affair person actually did together. For some people, assessing the potential social threat is also important. Learning of a partner's affair is shocking enough.

What Happened?

- When did the affair begin? Is this person someone you've known for a while? How long had you been feeling attracted to the other person prior to the affair? When did the relationship first become flirtatious? When did it become sexual (if it was sexual)?

- Who initiated the affair? Did either one of you try to stop it? If so, how? What prevented those efforts from working?

- Is the other person married or in a committed relationship? Does that person's partner know? If so, what was the partner's response? If not, do you or the affair person intend to tell the other partner?

- When and where did you get together? How long did the affair last? How many times did you and the other person engage in sexual activity?

- How much emotional involvement was there? How frequently did you and the outside person talk with or write to each other? What else did you do together?

- What kinds of contraception or protection against sexually transmitted diseases (STDs) were used? Did you sometimes not use protection? Have you or the other person been tested for STDs?

- How much money was spent on the affair? Were gifts exchanged? What do you intend to do with gifts or other mementos from the affair?

- Has the affair ended? If so, when and why? Who ended it? If the affair has ended, is this just for now or permanently? What contact have you had with the outside person since then? What steps, if any, have you taken to ensure that no further contact takes place? What does the outside affair person want? What are your plans if the outside person contacts you first?

- Who else knows about the affair? What do others know, and how did they find out?

- Are there any other consequences we need to consider? Could there be any complications at work or other legal problems? Could the outside person make our lives more difficult if she wanted to? Could the outside person's partner cause more difficulties? Are we in physical danger?

The last thing you need on top of that is to worry about who knows what and who is talking about you behind your back or to be blindsided by an outsider's comments.

Of course, there may also be actual physical threats that need to be considered. Foremost among these is the risk of STDs. If unprotected sex occurred, both of you should be evaluated medically for risks or indications of an STD. Separate from issues of risk for disease are threats of physical violence. We've worked with couples in situations where the outside affair person reacted to the unwanted ending of an affair by becoming physically aggressive toward either the participating or injured partner. On occasions, the outside person's own partner has become aggressive toward the participating partner. We're not proposing undue alarm, but we do suggest a candid and realistic discussion of potential physical aggression or other forms of retaliation from anyone involved in the affair, either directly or indirectly.

What couples should avoid discussing are the "gory" intimate details of the affair—especially in terms of specific sexual behaviors. Tom's insistence that Pam disclose everything she and her affair partner did in bed together didn't bring him emotional security; it didn't make him feel better about Pam, himself, or their marriage. Instead, it made it even harder for Tom to replace images of the affair in his mind with more helpful visions of times when he and Pam had been at their best together, or of how they could reach that state again.

Of course, knowing what matters need to be discussed isn't always enough to ensure productive conversations. Like Pam and Tom, you might find that you and your partner end up mired in frustrating cyclical harangues that leave you both with mounting frustration and resentment. If that's the case, turn to Chapter 3, where we offer guidelines for talking about feelings productively—and for listening well too.

Why Did You Do It?

Gaining a full understanding of how the affair came about is critical to regaining a sense of security and making good decisions about how to move on. So you may be surprised to see that the box on page 36 contains so few items. This isn't because we consider this question unimportant or expect it to be "in the background" following the initial discovery or disclosure of an affair. It's often the most consuming question that injured partners have. However, prolonged, detailed discussions about why the affair occurred aren't likely to be very productive or satisfying at this time. One reason is that the participating partner often doesn't really *know* why. Later in the recovery process we've heard, "I must have been crazy. What on earth was I thinking?" and "At first I didn't really understand how it came about. I thought I did—but the more I looked at things, the more I realized that most of my initial assumptions about why I had the affair were wrong." Pushing for conclusive answers now will likely produce only inaccurate or incomplete explanations, which can get in the way of looking more closely at the bigger picture later on.

Another reason that probing for "Why?" is often unproductive is that your partner knows that no explanation is likely to calm or satisfy you and therefore doesn't want to talk about it. For most people, nothing justifies a partner's having an affair, and so no "reason" suffices. Your partner may also sincerely want to avoid causing you further pain by discussing her own relationship unhappiness or disappointments. Some people who have an affair also feel ashamed to the point of genuine pain, and persistent questions about "why" only exacerbate this by forcing them to revisit the conclusion that there *was* no decent rationale or explanation for what they did.

Why Did You Do It?

- Why do you think the affair happened? What was going on with you? What else was going on in your life? What was going on between us?
- What were you thinking about me and our family?
- Why didn't you tell me? (or, Why did you wait to tell me?)

So, rather than suggesting that you avoid the "why" questions entirely, we advise you to avoid spending endless hours going over the same questions. Some couples literally exhaust themselves staying up talking night after night and still feel they're getting nowhere. Part II of this book is devoted to examining how the affair came about; try to be patient and wait until you've read through Part I before pushing for full answers to these questions.

Where Does This Leave Us?

Where the affair will leave you in the long run is uncertain, but for now you need to establish boundaries defining your current interactions, including how to deal with basic tasks and what kinds of contact to have. Common questions addressing these concerns are listed in the box on page 37. Some of these—for example, how to deal with daily family and household responsibilities and how to express emotional or physical closeness—need to be addressed early on. Others—for example, considerations of separation or divorce—are better dealt with later unless one of you has already taken steps in this direction. In short, try to distinguish between immediate decisions that need to be made *now* and those that will be better informed *later*, after you've taken time to work through the step-by-step process of exploring how the affair occurred and how to move on outlined in Parts II and III of this book.

Among the more important issues you might be debating is whether to continue living together. **In general, we usually advise couples _not_ to**

Where Does This Leave Us?

- What about us? Should we continue to live together?
- Have you considered divorce? What steps, if any, have you already taken? Have you talked with anyone about moving in with him or her? Have you contacted an attorney? Have you set up a separate bank account?
- How do we make sure that we talk about the things that need to be talked about? Should we set limits on how long we talk at any one time or what we say to each other? How should we handle it when our discussions start to get out of control?
- How do we deal with the basic tasks of managing the relationship and our household? Do we continue to do laundry together, cook meals, or clean up afterward together? Go to church or the kids' ball games together?
- What acts of caring feel okay right now? Should we still call each other during the day just to chat? Do we still have our morning coffee together?
- What other expressions of intimacy do we want? Is it okay to touch one another or to hold hands? Are hugs okay? Do we still sleep together? Do kisses feel okay? What about making love together? What do we do if it starts to feel uncomfortable for either one of us?
- What do you think it would take for us to get through this? How willing are you to make these changes, and for how long?
- What commitments, if any, does either of us feel prepared to make at this time? Are we ready to make commitments about this relationship in the short term? About how to work toward moving on? About our own relationships with our children?
- Do you know what you want in the long run? How did you reach that decision, and how certain are you that your feelings won't change?

---

separate during the initial stages of dealing with an affair unless they absolutely can't remain together for the time being. Reestablishing a sense of security in your relationship is often vital to recovery, and separation can make this accomplishment more difficult. In addition, you and your partner will need to discuss many issues in order to move on successfully, and separating before you do so can make it more difficult to talk about them later. If you have children, a separation may not be in their best interest. Separating sometimes encourages the outside affair partner to pursue the participating partner even more aggressively, which usually deepens the wounds rather than healing them. Finally, separating may serve as a public announcement of the affair, which can lead to other complications, discussed in Chapter 4. Under certain circumstances it may be a good idea to separate, however; see the box below.

When a Separation Following an Affair Is a Good Decision

- *When one of you is absolutely certain of your decision to pursue a divorce.* It may be easier to separate now and move ahead with the divorce process, but please be cautious. What seems certain now may not seem as clear just a few weeks ahead.
- *When you can't avoid repeated intense and verbally aggressive arguments* (even using the strategies in Chapter 3). Separating for now may be your last resort for not making things worse.
- *When the emotional turmoil in your relationship is contributing to physical aggression*—pushing, restraining, slapping, or worse.

Related to the issue of a separation, you each need to know whether the other has taken any steps to pursue a divorce. *Thoughts* about divorce aren't uncommon at times like this. But if either partner has consulted an attorney or has recently set up separate financial accounts, it's important that the other partner be informed of this in order to be aware of what's happening. Part of the damage from an affair is the secrecy and deceit; don't make things worse by taking other strong actions that your partner doesn't know about. The goal at this point isn't to "win." Rather, the goal is to ensure that whatever long-term decisions you reach, you're each able to move on with dignity and without hurting one another or others you care about.

Each of you should tell the other what you want broadly, now, in terms of the relationship. That doesn't necessarily mean deciding what you want to do about your relationship in the long run. By and large, we think that most couples often aren't prepared to make definite long-term decisions because they don't yet have all the information they need. Instead, we're talking here about short-term decisions concerning the relationship. Do you each want to consider the possibility of making it work? Are you each prepared to commit to a process of examining how the affair came about and what it means for you both in the long run? Can you enter this process together?

How Can We Start to Return to Normal?

For Heidi and Ted, everything felt awkward after Ted confessed his affair. Heidi described it as "walking on broken glass" because they had to treat each other so gingerly. They knew they couldn't continue in their relationship like this, but they weren't sure how to take even the first steps toward getting back on track.

Once you decide whether you're going to continue living together, you may need to discuss how to handle matters that you no longer deal with automatically. Among them are tasks that just keep the relationship or family moving along. You need to look at what daily tasks have been disrupted by the affair and decide how they'll be carried out now. Will you divide up household responsibilities—laundry, house care, child care, bill paying—as you did before? Can you still do any of these tasks jointly? Can you handle them exclusively when they benefit both of you? If not, can you agree on a new system for getting things done so that neither one of you is hurt further and your relationship doesn't experience more damage? Exercise 2.2 will help you answer these questions.

Then there are the acts of caring that now feel so awkward. Maybe you used to phone each other during the day just to chat, or reconnect after dinner by taking a walk and discussing each other's day. You may have exchanged small gestures, such as offering to get each other something from the kitchen before bedtime or suggesting that you rent a movie and watch it together. Retreating into sustained silence for days or weeks on end can eat away at the foundation of your relationship. By contrast, finding a way to continue some of the previous acts of caring says, "I know things may not be resolved. I know there's still hurt and tension between us. But I'm doing this to let you know that I still care, and I'm not giving up yet." When couples aren't able to engage in "joint" activities such as playing games together or going out to dinner where conversation is expected, we encourage "parallel" activities that allow you to be together without requiring a lot of interaction—perhaps watching a movie together or attending a sporting event or theater production together. You need to strike a balance here. Make an effort to be thoughtful and considerate, but also recognize that you may not be comfortable right now with some of the ways you've shown love or affection in the past.

Finally, deciding how to handle intimate aspects of your relationship, including both sex and physical affection, can be particularly difficult. Are you each comfortable with gentle touches? Tender hugs or passionate kisses? Are you ready to sleep together? If you've stopped making love, are you ready to become sexually intimate again? We've seen people differ tremendously in their preferences along these lines. For some couples, making love following an affair can be a genuine means of reconnecting and comforting one another, while still acknowledging that parts of the relationship feel very uncertain or confusing. For other couples, even gentle touches can feel uncomfortable or a violation of personal boundaries during this chaotic time. We don't advocate any one way of dealing with this area over another. What's important is that you and your partner discuss this in ways that aren't demanding or hostile. Decisions you make in the short run won't prevent you from reaching different decisions down the road. Moreover, you should anticipate fluctuations in how either one of you feels about emotional or sexual intimacy, particularly the injured partner. What feels comfortable and soothing today may feel awkward or even traumatic tomorrow, and vice versa. Probably the best way to find out what your partner wants is to ask. Too often people try to read each other's body language and misinterpret what the other person wants. Such misunderstandings can escalate quickly when they're not checked with direct questions: "When I touched you last night, you pulled back from me. Would you rather I not touch you at all?"

Why Do Things Sometimes Suddenly Fall Apart? Coping with Flashbacks

If setting boundaries is the most important way to avoid making things worse, learning to cope with flashbacks comes in a close second. When you and your partner seem to be doing better and things suddenly fall apart, it's easy to feel as if you've erased everything you learned—and then some.

> *Jack and Barbara were driving along the highway on their way to a nearby resort for the weekend, amiably chatting about Barbara's work. They felt good about the progress they'd made in working to recover from Barbara's affair a few months ago, and both had really looked forward to this getaway together.*
>
> *Suddenly Jack stopped talking, and when Barbara turned toward him she noticed he was gripping the wheel tightly and his expression was grim. What had she said that had upset him? When she asked him what was wrong, Jack said they'd just driven by a motel of the same chain where Barbara and her affair partner had sometimes gone in their hometown. Seeing another motel of the same name had made Jack feel sick to his stomach all over again.*
>
> *Barbara instantly felt plunged into despair. They would never recover, no matter what she did. She couldn't control Jack's reactions and would never be able to see these mood swings coming. And why did he have to bring up her affair, at this of all times? Why did he have to ruin the weekend for them? What did he expect from her? She couldn't eliminate all the motels in the world that might remind him of her affair. Why couldn't he just agree to move on?*

Jack and Barbara's struggles with reminders of her affair demonstrate an inevitable part of the recovery process. Driving by a motel of a similar name, seeing a car of the model owned by the outside person, answering the phone only to have the caller hang up can all trigger memories of those deeply painful, traumatic feelings that accompanied the discovery of a partner's affair. And besides the personally relevant details that evoke flashbacks, TV, newspapers, and movies are filled with references to infidelity. Reexperiencing the affair, even when both partners are convinced that the affair has ended, often occurs at unpredictable times and is nearly always deeply distressing for both.

We're going to emphasize here the kinds of acutely distressing flashbacks frequently experienced by injured partners. But it's important to understand that participating partners can also struggle with memories that evoke guilt, shame, or even sometimes feelings for the outside person, and

41

that the guidelines offered on the next few pages may be helpful for dealing with these as well.

How Can I Recognize When I'm Having a Flashback?

In the strictest sense, *flashback* refers to a reexperiencing of a traumatic incident with the same emotional, cognitive, and physiological reactions felt at the time the trauma occurred. But if you think of flashbacks as occurring along a continuum, with true reexperiencing at one end and experiences more like rueful memories at the other, flashbacks related to affairs fall somewhere in the middle. The memories are painful enough to disrupt your thoughts and feelings, but you're fully aware that the trigger is distinct from the event itself. Flashbacks at any level involve painful feelings, memories, and images from the past. Because they occur suddenly and unexpectedly, they typically feel unpredictable and beyond your control.

Flashbacks usually are very upsetting to both partners. But they can become even more distressing when misunderstood or mismanaged. Often, the participating partner concludes that the injured partner is experiencing the flashback intentionally, unwilling to let go, or using the flashback experience to punish him. The injured person can feel frightened, overwhelmed, and hopeless about ever getting over it. Therefore, unless you and your partner develop an effective way of recognizing and responding to flashbacks, they may be a real setback to your progress and ultimately block your recovery. Guidelines for coping with flashbacks are summarized in the box on page 43. Exercise 2.3 at the end of this chapter will help you and your partner use these guidelines in developing specific strategies for dealing with flashbacks.

If you're having flashbacks, you need to decide on when and how to share these. Following the initial discovery of an affair, you'll probably experience many reminders that trigger sadness, hurt, or anger. However, asking your partner to discuss with you *every* memory you have of the affair, or every reexperiencing no matter what the level of intensity, can eventually wear your partner down. So try to evaluate the importance of discussing your flashback in any given situation. If your memory or flashback is highly distressing to you and you need support, if it's interfering with your ability to interact constructively with your partner, or if your partner asks about your feelings during a flashback, you should probably discuss it. But sometimes it will be important for

Guidelines for Coping with Flashbacks

- If you recognize that you're responding to your partner in a panicky, worried, accusatory, or angry manner, step back and evaluate the situation and your reaction.

- If you decide that your reaction is realistic given the immediate circumstances, express your feelings to your partner and work to find a more acceptable solution to this problem. For example: *"When you're an hour late getting home from work and haven't called, it makes me worry about where you are, and who you're with or what you're doing—just like I used to right after your affair. I'd like us to agree on how to handle occasions when you get delayed unexpectedly."*

- If you decide that your reaction is most likely a reaction to a memory of the affair, let your partner know what is happening by describing your feelings and linking them to the memory that has been activated. For example: *"Driving by that motel just triggered memories of your affair, and I feel hurt and frightened all over again."*

- Try to distinguish among the different feelings you're having and how aroused you're becoming physically. For example: *"When the phone just rang while we were sleeping, I flashed back to when he used to call you late at night during your affair. It felt like it was happening all over again. My heart is pounding. It feels just as intense as it did back then."*

- Be specific about what would be most helpful at this moment in dealing with these feelings. Do you simply want your feelings to be understood and acknowledged? Do you want your partner to respond to your feelings by offering to hold you, reassure you, or provide you time and space to be by yourself? For example: *"I've been feeling more alone and distant from you today. I really need you to be with me and just hold me for a while."*

- Work with your partner to find ways to reduce the likelihood or frequency of these triggers happening again. For example: *"Watching movies together used to be fun, but right now I really need us to avoid movies about romance, infidelity, or other reminders of your affair. How can we manage that?"*

- Balance discussions with your partner about flashbacks with efforts to deal with these experiences on your own to avoid overwhelming your relationship or wearing down your partner with these difficult interactions.

you to try to cope with these experiences on your own. In balancing your efforts to cope with flashbacks as a couple versus dealing with them on your own, use some of the self-care strategies described in Chapter 5.

How Should I Respond to My Partner's Flashbacks?

Participating partners need to know how to respond to the injured partner's flashbacks without making things worse. If you think your partner may be experiencing a flashback or other emotional reaction to memories of your affair, ask if this is so and invite your partner to share his or her feelings with you. Your partner may prefer not to talk with you about it. If so, try to accept that decision for now. More likely, your partner will interpret your offer as your willingness to listen to his or her feelings in an effort to offer support or understanding. Use the guidelines for effective listening discussed in Chapter 3. Describe specifically what you're observing in your partner without attacking and ask your partner to label his or her feelings: "You seem quiet all of a sudden, and you look pretty tense. Do you want to talk about what's going on?"

Try to help your partner identify the trigger (or triggers) for what he or she is currently feeling. Is it something you've said or done without realizing it? Was it some other trigger in the environment? Was it something inside your partner—such as thinking about how he or she didn't measure up to the outside person and suddenly seeing an image of the other person? When your partner identifies the trigger, try to avoid becoming defensive. For example, if your partner describes experiencing an acute flashback when the phone rings and an anonymous caller hangs up, that doesn't mean your partner believes you're having an affair all over again. You don't need to defend yourself, repeatedly assert that you're no longer having an affair, or insist that your partner stop having such thoughts. Instead you can respond, "I'm sorry this happened to you. I know it feels terrible. We'll get through it together." Try to listen and be caring; it doesn't mean you've just done something wrong.

In addition to clarifying the particular trigger at the moment, consider talking about the things that tend to trigger such intense feelings for each of you. Identifying these triggers can help both of you recognize high-risk situations. In some cases, you can rearrange things to avoid likely triggers—for example, avoid staying late at work alone. Some triggers can't always be avoided, but recognizing triggers in advance can help you reduce their occurrence and manage their impact more effectively.

What Can I Do to Help Right Now?

Inviting your injured partner to describe what he wants from you in this moment can help the two of you work together to deal with these difficult experiences. Anticipate that your partner's desires may change across different situations. Usually there's nothing you can do to "fix it." Often what the injured partner needs is some form of support while experiencing these strong feelings. Sometimes your partner might want to be held and reassured that you care and will be there for him; other times your partner may want to talk and express his feelings. Sometimes she might want to have a problem-solving discussion and decide how to avoid certain triggers—for example, finding a different driving route to avoid certain motels. Other times, your partner might want to be alone to try to relax and get away from the feelings or just to cry. And still other times your partner may not be sure what he wants or may say one thing at first and feel differently later. So be patient and try to remain flexible. If your partner initially asks to be left alone, check back again later and see if her feelings have changed and she now prefers to have you nearby. Most important is that you approach these flashbacks as a couple. First clarify whether your partner is having some type of flashback experience so there are no misunderstandings; then talk about what your partner needs and what you can do right now to be helpful.

What Should We Expect Regarding These Setbacks?

For now you should probably anticipate that flashbacks at various levels of reexperiencing might continue for a while, particularly if you're the injured partner and you've recently learned about the affair. You should also probably expect that just when these experiences seem to be behind you, they'll pop up again in ways that may feel discouraging. Flashbacks can be painful and can cause either you or your partner to fear that recovery will never occur. But flashbacks don't mean that you're back to square one, your partner isn't trying, or the situation is hopeless. Flashbacks are a typical part of the recovery process. In our experience, flashbacks gradually diminish in frequency, intensity, and traumatic impact on both partners and the relationship. You can facilitate this process by staying hopeful, working together, and using the guidelines outlined here.

What's Next?

Do the following exercises and then go on to Chapter 3, where we'll help you develop more effective ways of expressing and responding to each other's feelings, make decisions together, and lower the temperature during heated discussions. Because so many of these skills and strategies are helpful in dealing with the matters discussed in this chapter, many people find it helpful to read Chapters 2 and 3 together to consider how to integrate skills from Chapter 3 into their Chapter 2 work. You can always come back to the Chapter 2 exercises and then read Chapter 3 in full.

——————————— Exercises ———————————

The following exercises are designed to help you and your partner deal with challenges in interacting. It's best to do them together, but we give instructions here for doing them separately too.

• *If you're working with your partner:* First read through the exercises separately and write down your individual responses. Then schedule a time to exchange and discuss your responses. Limit any discussion to 30 minutes even if that means discussing only one question or part of a question—better to do that effectively than to rush through the questions or spend too much time and end up tired, discouraged, or hurt. You're more likely to come back and try again if you can keep your discussions constructive.

• *If you're working through this book separately or alone:* Read through the exercises on your own and write down your individual responses. Consider whether your partner might be willing to sit down with you and talk about the issues addressed. If so, agree on a time when you're both willing to give 15–30 minutes to begin considering these issues one at a time. The more constructive you can make these initial discussions, the more likely your partner may be to engage in more difficult discussions down the road. Use the exercises to decide how *you* would like to interact with your partner. Focus on your own behaviors. Regardless of where you two end up, you're likely to feel better about yourself if you can look back and know that you managed your own behaviors as well as possible.

EXERCISE 2.1. TALKING ABOUT THE AFFAIR

This first exercise is designed to help you and your partner manage difficult initial discussions about the affair. But if you're already having trouble with discussions spiraling out of control, skip ahead to Chapter 3 to get help with devising strategies to deal with this.

What to Talk About

Your discussions are likely to go better if you can limit the number of questions you present to your partner at this time and make your questions as specific as possible. *List the top five questions you'd most like to talk with your partner about at this time.* Try to focus on information you need to have now to get through the next few weeks. For example:

"When did the affair begin and end?"

"Was there ever a time when you didn't use protection against a sexually transmitted disease?"

"Have you already decided to end our relationship?"

Avoid the "why" questions as much as possible for now. We'll get to these important questions at a later time. To keep the discussion from being one-sided, you might consider asking your partner to list the top few questions that he or she would like to ask you.

When and Where to Talk About It

Your discussion will probably go better if you and your partner agree on when, where, and for how long to have your first few discussions. *Write down your proposal for when and where to have your initial discussions with your partner about the affair. Share this proposal with your partner and try to reach a specific agreement. If your partner doesn't agree with your initial proposal, explore other possibilities.* For example:

"Let's sit down for 30 minutes Tuesday evening in the living room after the children go to bed to begin discussing my top five questions. During that time, we agree not to answer the phone or the door. After 30 minutes, regardless of where we are, we'll stop for the night and continue another time."

EXERCISE 2.2. DECIDING HOW TO INTERACT FOR NOW

Many areas of the relationship, from handling chores to physical intimacy, may feel confusing or uncertain to you or your partner right now. It's important to work toward decisions that specify what each partner will and will not do and what the trial period will be, such as the next few days or the next few weeks.

If you and your partner get stuck and find yourselves unable to reach tentative decisions in the areas emphasized below, you may want to draw on the specific guidelines for decision making discussed in Chapter 3.

Managing Basic Tasks

You and your partner probably need to reach decisions about a variety of chores. *List the top five tasks or areas of responsibility that you and your partner will need to decide how to handle in order to get through the next week or two. For each of these (1) state what the task or concern is, clearly and specifically, and (2) propose some possible solutions.* For example:

"We need to decide how to handle the kids' activities after school. I propose that we continue the same transportation plans we've used in the past. I'd like us both to continue to attend their events and sit together, but without the need to talk with each other if we don't feel like it."

Or

"I'd like us to continue to have meals together at night, but for the time being not to have lunch together anymore."

Or

"I'd like you to continue to pay the bills, but I'd like a brief update every week on what's been paid out and what our bank balance is so I can be better informed about our finances."

Engaging in Acts of Caring

In the past, you and your partner may have exchanged simple acts of caring that now feel uncertain or awkward—for example, calling on the phone during the day just to chat, going for a walk together, offering a neck massage, or making the other person a snack. *List four or five ways that you'd like you and your partner to engage in simple acts of caring over the next few weeks. As you list these, try to include one or two behaviors in each of these categories:*

- *Unilateral: Things either of you can do on your own for the other.* For example:

  "I'd like you to check over my car for me at the beginning of each week to make sure I have enough gas and that the oil and tires are okay."

- *Parallel: Things you do together but that don't require much interaction.* For example:

  "I'd like us to watch a movie together."

  Or

  "I'd like us to go to church together."

- *Joint: Things that you do together that involve direct interaction.* For example:

  "I'd like to go to dinner with you and just enjoy ourselves, with no discussion of what happened. I need some time together that feels relaxed and safe."

Dealing with Your Sexual Relationship

You and your partner need to decide how you're going to deal with your physical or sexual relationship over the next few weeks. Your feelings about this may change over time, so it will be important to have a strategy for how to check back with each other on this from time to time. Because the two of you may have different preferences concerning your level of sexual involvement right now, the guideline we encourage is to limit these exchanges to the safest level needed by either partner. *List the level of physical or sexual involvement that you would like to have with your partner over the next week or two. Describe who you'd like to be responsible for initiating these interactions and how you'd like to handle it if either one of you becomes uncomfortable during these times. For example:*

> "Sometimes I need us to make love because it feels reassuring to me. Other times I'm not comfortable even with your just touching me. I'd like for either one of us to be able to give the other a simple hug outside of the bedroom. But, for now, to feel safe I want to be the one to initiate anything more than that—including making love or even kissing. If we're beginning to become more intimate and it starts to feel uncomfortable for me, I want to be able to say so and for us to stop what we're doing without any explanation required and without either of us getting angry toward the other."

> Or

> "For right now, I really don't want any physical contact. I just can't handle it; it brings everything right back. So let's not touch each other for now but check back with each other in a week or two."

EXERCISE 2.3. COPING WITH FLASHBACKS

Because flashbacks are so common following an affair and can interfere with recovery, it's important for you and your partner to try to understand how they come about and develop plans for coping with them.

Recognizing a Flashback

Try to recall different times when you suddenly found yourself thinking about the affair at an unexpected time or place. What thoughts were you having? What feelings were you experiencing? What bodily sensations did you have, such as muscle tension, shortness of breath, or a sick feeling in your stomach? Or try to recall times when you became aware that your partner was experiencing a flashback linked to the affair. How did you become aware of this experience? What did your partner do or say? What did you observe on your own? *Describe as many signs or aspects of your own or your partner's flashback experiences as you can identify.*

Identifying Triggers

Try to identify as many triggers as possible for the flashback experiences you recalled in the previous step. Where were you, and where was your partner? What was each of you doing? What was happening before and at the time of the flashback? The more specifically you can identify triggers of flashbacks, the more you and your partner may be able to minimize their happening. If you were with your partner and became aware of a sudden change in his or her mood that seemed unrelated to what was happening between the two of you, can you recall what else was going on at the time? Has your partner ever described triggers for painful reexperiencing of the affair? *Describe as many triggers for your own or your partner's flashback experiences as you can identify.*

Coping with Flashbacks

Try to develop as many ways of coping with flashbacks as you can. Some of these should be for you together as a couple; others should be for the person experiencing the flashback to cope with on his or her own.

Explore strategies for you and your partner to cope with flashbacks together. For example, how can you let your partner know if you're experiencing a flashback? Or if your partner's mood or behaviors suddenly change in ways that confuse you that you believe may be linked to a flashback, how can you ask about it in a way that reflects your concern and willingness to help? Once you're both aware that one of you is experiencing a flashback, what steps can you take to reduce the duration or impact of this experience? What responses from the partner would be most helpful—both in that moment and following? For example, if the person experiencing the flashback initially wants separate time and space alone, should the other partner still check back later to see whether this need has changed to a wish for closeness and reassurance? When and how would you each like that approach to be pursued?

Similarly, identify ways for you to cope with flashbacks on your own. For example, does redirecting your thoughts and energies to other activities help to minimize thoughts and feelings linked to the affair? Does this strategy work better when you engage in individual activities by yourself, such as reading, going for a walk, pursuing a hobby, or engaging in exercise? Or do you find you can more effectively redirect your thoughts and energies by engaging with others, such as spending time with your children, another family member, or a close friend? Do you find meditation, prayer, or spiritual or inspirational reading helpful in gaining a sense of calm or redirection in your life? For each of these individual strategies for coping with flashbacks, identify any assistance you may need from your partner, such as providing an opportunity to be by yourself or help in watching the children while you engage in self-care. If you have difficulty thinking of strategies for coping with flashback experiences on your own, turn to Chapter 5 for suggestions on how to care for yourself better.

3

>>> ——————————————————————————

How Do We Talk
with Each Other?

When Bill discovered that Mary was having an affair with a customer at work, what happened followed a familiar pattern: Bill threatened divorce, and Mary broke off the brief affair almost immediately. They argued constantly, and Bill planned to move out. When he was starting to pack his bags, they both realized they weren't ready to end their 10-year marriage. Mustering all their energy and more reason than they felt they had, they pulled back from the brink and found ways to limit their verbal battles. They forced themselves to continue family meals, to go to the kids' soccer games together, to figure out who would drive the kids where and who would handle the grocery shopping and laundry for the week. Grim but functioning, they got through the first few weeks.

It didn't take long, however, for Mary and Bill to become painfully aware of the emptiness in what had once been a full and close relationship. They were sleeping in the same bed but not making love. When they tried to talk about the affair and their relationship, neither could seem to find the right words to be understood. Bill had never felt more profoundly alone in his life. He couldn't imagine being able to restore the closeness he and Mary had once enjoyed, but he also couldn't imagine living without her. When he tried to explain to Mary that he felt wounded at a depth he had never experienced before, and why at times he still froze when she touched him, he just ended up repeating how hurt he was. In response, Mary kept saying that she understood and was sorry for what she had done.

But Bill didn't feel understood, and Mary didn't know what else to say. How many times and how many different ways could she say she was sorry? She knew Bill was devastated, but saying she understood seemed to have little impact. She believed it was her role to listen, but at times it hurt to do so. Seeing the contempt in his eyes made her wince. And it hurt when she felt his pain, knowing she had caused it. Mary also struggled with her own hurt. For several years she had tried to tell Bill how shut out she felt from his life. His life revolved around his work. She had no longer felt important to him. She knew this feeling had partly led to her looking for support and attention elsewhere. It was no excuse for her affair, but it had been a factor. Still, there was just no way she could tell Bill this—not after what she had done. Yet, until he understood, how could they really begin to rebuild their relationship?

Eventually Bill grew tired of trying to explain how he felt, and Mary seemed tired of trying to understand.

Feeling understood by your partner is one of the most important parts of an intimate relationship. Two people don't marry just because they can get along with each other without arguing. They also don't usually marry simply because they share common interests. Most people enter into a long-term committed relationship because they feel special to each other. They often feel uniquely understood—able to talk about deep feelings and disclose parts of themselves that they ordinarily wouldn't share with anyone else. When the relationship is working well, there's an underlying foundation of trust and security. The ability and opportunity to share deep feelings, to have these feelings heard and understood, and to experience warm and tender caring form the very core of intimacy.

An affair shatters this foundation, especially for the injured partner. The person you counted on most to be caring, to avoid causing you pain, to be faithful, to provide support when life is most difficult is no longer reliable. The future of the relationship seems in doubt. It no longer feels safe to express feelings that make you vulnerable. Being hurt definitely makes you feel vulnerable, so much of your hurt is transformed into anger or rage. Sometimes the shock and pain are so profound that you become numb just to get through the day. At other times, the anger turns inward and combines with doubts about your own adequacy or attractiveness to produce a deep depression. Anger and depression, fight and flight, attack and withdrawal may alternate in rapid or unpredictable ways. In the midst of this chaos, the ability to express yourself clearly, in a way that can be heard and understood by your partner, is as difficult as it is vital.

If you're the participating partner, you may very well be struggling with your own feelings of disappointment or hurt, which may interfere with your ability to listen and respond effectively to your partner's feelings.

In this chapter, we'll suggest some better ways of communicating with your partner. We offer certain skills for expressing your feelings and for responding to your partner's feelings that can help your partner hear what you're trying to say and help you both *feel* heard and understood. When you both feel understood, you can take full advantage of the problem-solving skills described here too. And for the inevitable moments when discussions become too heated, we'll give guidelines for keeping them from escalating out of control.

Principles for Talking with Your Partner

When an affair has just been revealed, it's simply not reasonable to expect complete calm when you try to talk about it—or about anything, for that matter. It may help, however, to keep in mind three goals:

1. Keep the discussions balanced.
2. Keep them focused.
3. Prevent further damage.

These are effective principles for making conversations productive, but of course sticking to them can be difficult, which is why we offer specific tips for doing so first.

Keeping Balance

Balance is so elusive when hurt has been transformed into anger. One way to keep things from spinning out of control is to remember that the ultimate goal of your discussions with your partner is to find a way to move forward. When you focus only on what's bad—such as the participating partner's affair and its traumatic consequences—your discussions with

55

your partner can become too painful and disillusioning to continue. You'll get nowhere. Instead, try to acknowledge what was right with this relationship and what may be worth saving. However, this doesn't mean sugarcoating the past either. Don't "rewrite" the history of your relationship to make it sound all bad, and don't paint it as having been perfect until your partner ruined it with an affair.

Another way to keep the discussion balanced is to make sure both of you share your feelings and perspectives. Some participating partners believe they're obligated to sit quietly and put up with whatever the injured partner wants to say, and generally we do encourage participating partners to listen patiently and openly to their injured partner's distress. But we also know that over time intense criticism and verbal attacks, uninterrupted by anything positive, can erode whatever hope there is for working together toward recovery.

To move forward, you need to come to a good understanding of *each other's* perspective, by stepping back from your own feelings and trying to listen and speak to each other in a balanced way. Easier said than done, we know. But try to put yourself in your partner's shoes and see things from his or her perspective.

Staying Focused

Keeping your discussions focused means not allowing the affair to intrude into almost every moment of every interaction. Some couples have found it helpful to agree on a time and place to discuss concerns related to the affair—for example, at night after the children have gone to bed or in the morning after they've left for school. Others agree to a time limit on any one discussion—for example, 30 minutes maximum unless both partners agree that talking longer will be constructive. Some couples initially find it almost impossible to talk to one another without getting out of control. For them, writing down questions (no more than five at a time) and providing written responses (more than one or two words!) can be a way of expressing concerns and sharing information in a more controlled manner.

Keeping the affair from intruding is particularly critical at those times set aside for comfort or pleasure together. We've seen some tragic results when, for example, the injured partner asks the participating partner during lovemaking if that's how it was with the outside affair person. **Work hard at preventing painful discussions during such times.**

Another way to keep your discussions focused is to keep their content relevant to moving forward. For an injured partner, there's little that doesn't seem relevant to an affair. By contrast, for a participating partner, there's a *lot* that doesn't seem relevant. Anticipating this difference between the two of you might help you tolerate it a bit better and find a middle ground you can both live with for now. One way to keep your discussions relevant is to link whatever information you're seeking to specific steps or strategies for moving forward, such as "I want to know where you went out to dinner together, because for now I just don't think I could handle going to the same places with you. I want to be able to enjoy a dinner with you without thinking about her."

Preventing Further Damage

Avoiding making things worse may be the most important principle for discussing the affair. As explained in Chapter 2, preventing further damage is often a matter of establishing boundaries. In this case it means clarifying what you and your partner will discuss about the affair and in how much detail. In Chapter 2 we laid out the types of information that you'll want, and probably need, to get from your partner and what your partner should be willing to tell you. But where this issue of how much to ask and how much to tell causes the biggest problems is in how much explicit sexual detail the participating partner should reveal about the affair. Here is a specific area where we suggest you draw a clear line: ***Our recommendation is that you not discuss these details with each other.*** You need to know if your partner had intercourse with the other person, not specific details of who did what. Knowing more than that may create vivid mental images that will haunt you and make it even more difficult to move on.

If you find yourself obsessing over what your partner and the other person did in bed, know that most of the injured partners we've talked with who have ignored this caution have regretted it later. Especially if the affair was revealed very recently, your desire to hear the "gory details" may come from the belief that bringing the hidden parts of the affair out in the open will restore a sense of control to your life. Generally, we've found that knowing these details doesn't make people feel back in control at all. So we strongly encourage you to resist the impulse to insist on this kind of information. At the very least, hold off for now and see whether your desire for such information is as strong a few weeks or months down the road.

Talking about Feelings

How Can I Help My Partner Understand?

When you feel as if you've tried to convey the same message over and over, in many different ways, and still your partner doesn't understand, you can't help believing that your partner needs to listen and respond more effectively. And you may be right. But it's also possible that your message isn't as clear as you think or that one or both of you are making assumptions that aren't accurate. Using a few specific guidelines for expressing your feelings may send your message along a truer path. But first, here are some general guidelines for discussing feelings as a couple.

General Guidelines for Discussing Feelings as a Couple

• *Work to understand and respond to the other person's feelings before expressing your own.* How often do you find yourself preparing a response to your partner's comments before he's even finished speaking? If you think about it, you know that you do this at times, just like everyone else. But what you may not be aware of is that it's hard to really listen to the other person at the same time as you're thinking about what to say next.

• *Limit the feelings you're discussing to those that relate to a specific situation.* For example, if you're upset about something your partner said earlier in the day, don't allow the discussion to generalize to all the occasions when you've been upset over the past week.

• *If you reach a point where it's clear that either of you isn't communicating well, take a break until you can come back and try again.* Remember that talking about very deep and difficult feelings is perhaps the greatest challenge of recovering from an affair. Doing it well takes effort and practice. Doing it badly can inflict further damage and makes recovery more difficult.

• *Be clear with each other about* why *you're communicating.* Although there are many specific reasons for talking with your partner, most conversations are held to share ideas, thoughts, and feelings *or* to reach decisions or solve problems.

Sharing thoughts and feelings can help you feel connected, become more intimate, or get something off your chest. Conversations that focus on making decisions are more goal-oriented and answer the question

"What are we going to do?" Although both of these types of conversations are important—particularly for recovering from affairs—a common problem is that two partners can be pursuing different types of conversations at the same time. One partner merely wants to express feelings for the purpose of being understood or supported, and the other believes the goal is to reach a decision or solve a problem. When this mismatch occurs, both partners are likely to feel frustrated.

Keisha continued to feel sad and confused months after learning of Razi's affair. She was confident that his affair had ended. She had seen Razi's efforts to rebuild their relationship. They had struggled through the initial chaos and were working to make things better. But there were times when her deep hurt, doubts about herself, resentment toward Razi, and especially her worries about whether they would survive as a couple, washed over her. Razi could tell when she was struggling with these feelings. He typically asked what he could do to soothe them, reassure her, and help her get past her feelings. Keisha felt frustrated by his question. There wasn't anything he could do to make her feelings go away. She just wanted him to understand that sometimes she still hurt, and she still worried. Razi found Keisha's response equally frustrating. He had done everything she'd asked, and more. He felt completely ineffective in helping Keisha to resolve her feelings. What else could he do?

Keisha and Razi's dilemma is common among couples struggling to recover from an affair. It's common to continue to feel hurt, insecure, angry, or filled with despair long after learning of your partner's affair, and you need to express these feelings many times. And just as often, your partner searches for what else she can do to "fix" things to move the relationship forward and put the affair behind you.

Sometimes the challenge isn't to "fix" feelings but simply to understand them. Keisha learned that at those times it helped to begin the discussion by saying something like "Right now I just want you to understand what I'm feeling. I don't expect you to fix anything or do anything differently. But I've been feeling upset and alone, and I'd feel better if you at least understood what I'm experiencing."

At other times, Keisha needed more than understanding, but she still wasn't interested in making decisions or trying to solve problems. She was seeking care and reassurance, or time just to be by herself until she was able to get on top of her feelings and feel ready to interact with Razi again. At these times she would say something like "I'm feeling really anxious [or sad] again. It's not something to be solved. But right now I just need you to hold me, to tell me you love me, and that we'll continue to work through this together." Or instead she might say, "Razi, right now I'm upset and need some time for myself. It's not anything you've just done or not done. It's just that it's going to take time to get through this. For now, I just need an evening by myself, and I hope you can understand that."

Razi also became more skillful at distinguishing between discussions that involved decision making and those that simply required his listening and understanding. When Keisha didn't make it clear herself, he learned to ask: "I can tell you're upset, but I'm not sure what to do right now. Is this something we need to figure out how to deal with or do differently, or are you mostly just wanting me to listen to your feelings?" At other times after Keisha had expressed her feelings, Razi would ask what she wanted or needed from him. For example, he might say, "Keisha, I know you're upset right now about the affair. Do you want to still try to be together right now, or would you prefer some separate time for yourself?"

The specific language you use isn't important. What's important is that you make an effort to be clear about whether you're trying to resolve something or to communicate your thoughts and feelings.

- If you want a discussion about feelings, let your partner know that you're looking for understanding, not decision making.
- If there's a particular response to your feelings you're hoping for—for example, being comforted or having separate time for yourself—tell your partner what you want.
- If you're not sure whether your partner has started a discussion to share feelings or to resolve something or reach a decision, ask.

Specific Guidelines for Expressing Your Feelings

If discussions with your partner leave you feeling misunderstood, there are specific steps you can take to express your feelings in a way that may help your partner listen and understand. You might feel awkward using some of the guidelines that follow if they're not already part of your communication repertoire. But if you try to adapt them to fit your personal speaking style, they'll make discussions about feelings with your partner less difficult and more productive, and in turn they'll begin to feel more natural. You might pick out one or two that seem easiest to start.

• *Speak for yourself, not for your partner.* One way to do this is to use an "I" statement that links your feelings to a specific situation or behavior. Couple therapists refer to this as the "XYZ" formula, as in "When you do X in situation Y, I feel Z." For example, "When you tell me just to forget it when I'm asking you about your affair, I feel discounted and unimportant to you." Or, "When you ask me where I've been but then don't believe me when I tell you, I feel frustrated and no longer feel like trying to answer your questions." Another benefit of using this approach is that it will help you focus your feelings and tie them to specific situations, rather than expressing them as global and potentially more hurtful statements. It's easier for your partner to hear "It hurts me when we go to a party and you spend more time talking with others than with me" than "I feel unimportant to you because you never pay attention to me."

A second, equally important part of this guideline is *not* speaking for your partner. Many people have a tendency to tell a partner what the partner is thinking or feeling. Even if the speaker is correct, the listener usually resents it. So speak for yourself about your own thoughts and feelings and allow your partner to speak for him- or herself.

• *Express your feelings as your own subjective experience, not as absolute truths.* If you state your feelings as absolute truths, your partner is likely to take exception and tell you that you're wrong, proceeding to tell you the *"real"* truth. For example, think about what it's like to be on the receiving end of this statement: "You always ignore me." Now think about how different it feels to be on the receiving end of this statement: "When you don't talk with me when you come in from work, I feel ignored." The listener in the first case is almost sure to feel compelled to dispute the fact that he *always* ignores his partner, which means the conversation may never even get around to how his partner feels about feeling ignored. The listener in the second case is not being accused of always ignoring his partner, so he can more easily acknowledge the feeling—"I understand that's how you feel about it, and I respect that"—before considering, and discussing, whether a change in his own behavior is warranted.

• *Focus on your feelings before moving on to thoughts or opinions.* Feelings are less likely to bring about a rebuttal than thoughts or opinions that accompany them. If you say to your partner, "I've been feeling down much of the day," it's unlikely that your partner will respond with "No, you haven't." Your partner *might* respond with "I wish you could move on and be happy again." But most people will not presume to tell you how you do or don't feel. Once your partner responds with something like "Tell me more about that. What's going on with you?" you can describe the thoughts you've been having or situations that have contributed to your feelings.

Try to be as specific as possible in describing your feelings. Saying to your partner "I'm upset" isn't as specific as saying "I'm worried," "I'm discouraged," or "I'm annoyed." Similarly, saying "I feel better today" offers less information than "I feel more optimistic," "I feel more appreciated," or "I feel more energetic." If you find it difficult to find the right word to describe your feelings, referring to the list of common "feeling words" on page 63 might be helpful. Remember: The better able you are to describe specific feelings you're experiencing, the better your partner will be able to understand you.

• *When expressing negative feelings or concerns, also include any positive feelings you have.* Working at a balanced expression of both positive and negative feelings may make it more likely that your negative feelings will be heard and that your partner will be able to respond to them in a more understanding way.

> Following Maria's brief affair with one of her coworkers, Antonio was uncomfortable with some of the more revealing dresses that she wore to work. When he said, "I wish you wouldn't dress in such a provocative manner," she argued that many of the women at her office wore such outfits and she saw nothing wrong with it. Eventually, Antonio tried a more balanced approach: "Maria, you have a really nice figure. You work hard at keeping in shape and I'm proud of you for it. But I'd really prefer it if you would save some of those more revealing outfits for special occasions when you and I go out together. Your wearing that type of outfit to work makes me uncomfortable. It's not that I worry about you, but I don't want those guys salivating at my lovely wife." When he approached Maria in this way, she felt less criticized by Antonio and more willing to compromise.

Words for Describing Common Feelings

Positive Moods

Happy/Joyful	Cheerful	Excited	Delighted	Glad
	Pleased	Amused	Thrilled	
Close/Warm	Loving	Devoted	Sexy	Affectionate
	Secure	Tender		
Energy/Vigor	Active	Lively	Peppy	Adventurous
	Vigorous	Energetic	Friendly	Enthusiastic
Relaxed/Calm	Gentle	Peaceful	Contented	
Other Positive	Agreeable	Ambitious	Confident	Inspired
	Lucky	Fortunate		

Negative Moods

Depressed/Sad	Unhappy	Bored	Blue	Gloomy
	Grim	Discouraged	Low	Miserable
	Dejected	Hurt		
Anxious	Shaky	Tense	Restless	Nervous
	Fearful	Panicky	Insecure	Terrified
	Frightened	Worried	Shy	Confused
Angry	Frustrated	Resentful	Enraged	Furious
	Irritated	Disgusted	Outraged	Annoyed
Contemptuous	Critical	Disdainful	Hostile	
Fatigued	Exhausted	Tired	Listless	Sluggish
	Weary			
Other Negative	Bewildered	Lonely	Jealous	Guilty
	Ashamed			

• *Limit yourself to expressing one main feeling or idea at a time, and then give your partner an opportunity to respond.* When one person talks for a long time, the other often stops listening after a while. People have trouble staying focused when someone goes on and on. Restricting how long you talk in any one turn may, however, be one of the most challenging tasks you'll face in expressing your feelings. Limit yourself to just a few sentences, maybe five or six, and then give your partner a chance to respond. You'll have an opportunity to say more; just don't do it all at once. Then invite your partner to respond by asking something like "What do you think?" and wait *at least* 15 seconds or more before continuing if your partner remains silent. Some people need time to gather their thoughts before they respond. If your partner is one of those people, give your partner that time.

• *Choose your words and your timing carefully.* Work at using language that's specific and moderate in intensity. Negative statements that begin with "You always . . . " or "You never . . . " are rarely accurate and usually elicit a defensive response. Your partner is unlikely to accept judgments like "You're just not trustworthy." But she might respond more positively to "It's hard for me to trust you right now when you're out late and I don't know where you are."

Choosing when to talk can be as important as how you talk. Bringing up the affair as your partner is going to sleep or leaving the house for work doesn't allow time to discuss it. Moreover, for many people, the upset feelings linger during the day or interfere with falling asleep at night. Particularly if you're going to raise a difficult issue, try to do it when you're both available to have a thoughtful discussion.

Don't go to the opposite extreme either, holding hold back so long that your feelings build up inside until you finally explode because you can't take it anymore. To your partner it will seem as if you've merely overreacted to a minor incident. Brad had ended his affair months ago, but his flirtatious style with women really bothered Carmen. She didn't want to appear oversensitive, so she bit her tongue when he made joking, seductive comments to women at parties. Finally, one night when they got in the car at the end of the evening, she blasted him. Brad totally discounted her concerns because she seemed to have "lost it" over a simple joke to a woman, which he saw as totally innocent.

• *Accept responsibility for your own behaviors that may have contributed to the problem.* Rarely are problems in a relationship entirely one-sided. If you blame only your partner, your partner will likely defend himself and blame you back. Even if you believe your partner is responsible for 90% of a particular problem, search for the 10% of responsibility that is yours. The more you can demonstrate a willingness to accept ownership for your contributions to a problem, the easier it is for your partner to do so as well. It won't work perfectly every time, but with repeated efforts to share responsibility it's more likely that you and your partner can escape the mutual "blame game" and can each feel more understood.

How Can I Understand My Partner?

Effective communication requires equal parts of expressing your own feelings and listening and responding constructively to your partner. Being a good listener can be much harder than being a good speaker. How can you listen to and understand your partner, and how can you best *communicate* that understanding? You need to (1) communicate your willingness to listen up front, (2) respond appropriately while your partner is still speaking, and (3) respond constructively after your partner has finished.

Communicating Your Willingness to Listen

People who feel unheard are likely to respond in one of two ways. Your partner will either retreat and disengage from the conversation—"Why try if you're not going to listen?"—or try again to get the message across, perhaps repeating it in a louder voice or using more intense language. That is, people often escalate when they don't feel heard. It's as if they're saying, "If you didn't hear me, I'll tell you again louder and stronger, and maybe you'll get it this time!" You can help to avoid these problems by letting your partner know from the beginning that you're interested in understanding what your partner has to say.

You can effectively communicate your willingness to listen by adopting one of two strategies:

1. Making yourself available when your partner asks to be heard.
2. Inviting your partner to talk with you when he or she appears distressed.

Making yourself available means eliminating other distractions and offering your full attention. It can be as simple as turning to face your partner, making eye contact, and waiting to hear what your partner has to say. Or it can be more explicit—turning off the television, unplugging the phone, or moving to a place where you can both sit and face each other and saying, "What would you like to discuss?" Being available to listen is also communicated by how you present yourself nonverbally. Looks of impatience, an angry scowl, or arms tightly crossed all indicate an emotional resistance to listening. Instead, turn to your partner, relax your facial muscles, adopt a softened or more relaxed physical posture, and lower the volume of your voice when you respond.

Inviting your partner to talk with you when your partner appears distressed requires that you recognize that distress in the first place. Your partner may appear quieter than usual, less spontaneous or responsive to your touch, more irritable, or just more distracted. You can communicate your interest in listening by (1) checking out your partner's feelings, (2) offering to listen to these feelings, and (3) suggesting a time for talking further if necessary.

> When Beth noticed one evening that Mark seemed particularly quiet, she tried to pull him out of it by talking about her own day and asking about his, but he offered little in return. Finally she said, "You seem pretty quiet tonight, Mark, and I can't figure out what's going on. Are you upset about something?" Mark then told Beth that he had run into Charlie at a meeting and had found it almost unbearable as he recalled Beth's affair with Charlie that had ended six months earlier. Beth recognized that further discussion was important, but the timing was all wrong because the children were still up and demanding their attention. She responded to Mark's distress by saying, "I'm sorry. I know you're still upset. Could we talk about this some more after getting the children to bed?"

Responding While Your Partner Is Still Speaking

While your partner is speaking, *it's important to use body language to show you're still interested in listening.* Maintain eye contact, make your physical posture and facial expression receptive, and avoid scowling, foot tapping, and exasperated sighs. The following specific guidelines are also critical.

• *Don't interrupt.* Just as important as what you do nonverbally are things you say or don't say while your partner is speaking. Probably most important is listening without interrupting. Admittedly, it's hard to listen when your partner is talking about difficult issues, saying things that hurt you or that you disagree with. But your partner is unlikely to listen in the way you want before feeling heard and understood by you. One of you has to be willing to listen and demonstrate your understanding first, and we're encouraging you to be the one to do that.

- *Don't practice a rebuttal.* As your partner is talking, avoid preparing or rehearsing your response, a particular temptation when you already disagree with what your partner is saying. It's hard to listen and prepare a rebuttal at the same time. Your partner isn't going to feel heard if it's clear that you're anxiously awaiting your turn to speak, and if you *are* dying for your chance to talk, it's hard *not* to reveal your impatience through body language.

- *Avoid challenging, judging, and interpreting.* Avoid challenging your partner's feelings or views while listening. Avoid asking questions except to seek clarification. For example, it's okay to say, "I'm not sure I understand what you're saying. Could you tell me more about what you mean?" But it won't be helpful to say, "How could you feel that way? Tell me *why* you think that." In fact, as a general rule, "why" questions elicit more defensive or exaggerated statements as your partner feels obligated to justify her position. Similarly, avoid judging or interpreting your partner's thoughts and feelings while listening. Interpretations involve taking what your partner has said and giving it a different meaning. For example, if your partner is uncomfortable with the amount of time you spend with friends outside the home, refrain from making interpretations such as "There's really nothing wrong with my getting together with my friends. I think you've got this hangup that men can't be trusted."

- Finally, as you're listening to your partner and before you respond, be sure you *understand your partner's goal for this discussion.* Does your partner just want to be heard and understood, or does your partner want to solve a problem or reach a decision with you? If you're unsure, ask your partner to clarify. For example, "I'm not sure what you're looking for right now. Do you want to just sit and talk for a while about what you're feeling, or do you want us to make some decisions about what to do?"

Responding after Your Partner Has Finished Speaking

The best way to demonstrate that you've heard your partner is to repeat back the thoughts or feelings that your partner has expressed. Various terms describe this process: *mirroring, paraphrasing, reflecting,* and *active listening* are just a few. At the simplest level, you can demonstrate that you've accurately heard your partner by repeating or "parroting" what your partner has said, restating the message using your partner's original words: "I hear you saying you don't think we have sex often enough and you'd like us to change that." Although your partner still may not feel *understood* by you, it will at least be clear that your partner was *heard*.

A slightly higher level of responding involves restating your partner's thoughts or feelings in your own words by summarizing or paraphrasing what you've heard. The advantage to paraphrasing is that it demonstrates not only that you've literally "heard" your partner's words, but that you've understood them well enough to be able to express the same thought or feeling using alternative language. For example, "You'd like to make love more often, and you'd like us to explore ways of doing this together. Is that right?"

Sometimes your partner's feelings are only implied through tone of voice or body language. When this happens, you might demonstrate your understanding by labeling the implied feeling: "It sounds as though you're feeling frustrated that we're not making love as often as you'd like, and maybe you're feeling hurt that I don't appear as interested in you sexually as before. Is that right?" By checking out your reflection at the end with "Is that right?" you're inviting your partner to confirm or correct your understanding and also avoiding the appearance of mindreading or interpreting.

Some people are reluctant to paraphrase out of fear that doing so signals agreement. Reflecting isn't the same as agreeing—it's a way of letting your partner know that you listened and that you understand. And, in fact, one of the most important times to reflect is when you're about to disagree. Your partner will find it much easier to listen to your point of view if he has felt heard and respected by you. For example, you might say, "I know you're unhappy with our sex life right now, and you think I'm no longer sexually attracted to you. Is that right?" If your partner accepts your reflection, you might continue with "Actually, I'm very sexually attracted to you. That's part of the problem. When I start to feel attracted, I have these horrible thoughts about the affair that I can't get out of my mind. So I'm staying away not because I'm not interested in you—I just can't stand the terrible feelings that seem to come with it. I don't know how to get rid of those feelings."

Interestingly, research shows that happy couples don't paraphrase and validate very often during everyday conversations. Reflecting and validating aren't typical of our discussions when we're already feeling understood and feeling good about our relationship. But reflecting and validating may be essential when we're having trouble communicating in our relationships.

Active listening through reflection and validation can be very helpful when:

- Your partner isn't feeling understood by you.
- You want to ensure that your partner recognizes that you've heard and understood before offering your own contrasting thoughts or feelings.
- Your discussion is moving too quickly, escalating into an exchange of complaints and counter complaints. Reflections slow down the process.
- You're unsure of what your partner is trying to communicate, and you want to express your best understanding before asking for clarification.
- You want to focus on your partner's experience. Reflections keep the focus on what your partner has just said and invite your partner to continue sharing thoughts and feelings.

Reaching Decisions Together

Joel and Elsa kept going over and over their budget but could never agree on how to get their finances under control. Each discussion ended in a stalemate; Joel had his preferred solution, and Elsa had hers. Each seemed so intent on winning the argument that neither noticed they were losing the broader goal of finding a workable compromise to reduce their frequent quarreling over money. Their continuing bitterness began to seep into other areas of their lives.

How Do We Reach Decisions Together?

Even when you're doing well at listening and responding to each other's feelings, it's sometimes difficult to reach decisions together. You and your partner may easily get sidetracked. For example, if you're trying to decide whether to replace the washer, as you talked about last month, you might start to discuss how much extra money has already been spent because of the affair. Or the two of you may get deadlocked on an issue and find it difficult to compromise. Each of you may try to persuade the other of your own position, but there's no movement toward a middle ground. Or one of you tries to start a discussion about a recurrent problem in your relationship, but the other keeps retreating or avoiding the issue.

Having some concrete guidelines to rely on can be helpful at those times. These guidelines can apply whether the two of you are working to reach decisions together or you're struggling to reach individual decisions for yourself. When people are upset with each other and have trouble communicating, adding more structure to the conversation and following guidelines for reaching decisions can be especially helpful. We've found the following steps very helpful with couples in a variety of circumstances.

State the Issue without Blame

Often couples get off track because they're unclear about or have forgotten the specific issue they're trying to resolve.

> *Janet and Phil were struggling with what kinds of physical caring to exchange during the first month after Janet learned that Phil had ended a brief affair a few months earlier. Neither one felt good about not having any physical closeness, but they had difficulty identifying a comfort zone that felt right for both of them. When Phil tried to soothe Janet when he found her crying, she sometimes pushed him away. At other times, when he kept his distance when she was upset, she accused him of being cold and insensitive. Phil could have gotten angry in turn and accused Janet of being manipulative or impossible to please. Instead, Phil approached her and said, "Janet, I just don't know what you want right now or how to respond. I want to comfort you, but I don't want to make things worse by touching you when you don't want to be touched. We need to decide how we're going to handle physical affection and touching each other." Stating the issue clearly without anger and without blame brought it into the open and helped both of them look at the issue more constructively.*

Clarify Why the Issue Is Important

Partners don't always recognize or understand why an issue is important to the other person, so they don't have a good idea of what a good decision would be. For example,

> *Christy couldn't understand why Jim insisted that he didn't want his parents to know about Christy's affair. Christy thought Jim was trying to hide her affair from his parents because he was ashamed of her, and Jim thought Christy was insisting on telling his parents just to relieve her own conscience. Neither one understood the other until Jim clarified to Christy what his needs were and why this was important to*

him. He told Christy, "The reason I don't want to tell them right now is that I first want you and me to try to get our own relationship squared away. I'm afraid if we tell my parents, they'll never get over it, even if we stay together. I'm not ashamed of you; I just don't want to ruin your relationship with my parents. I think we'd be better off to wait a while and see what happens with us." This helped Christy to explain her own feelings and thoughts more effectively: "I'm not trying to make a confession to your parents just to help myself feel less guilty. But I want to reestablish my integrity so that, I hope, they can still have at least some level of respect for me, despite what I've done. I don't want to lie to them. But if you're suggesting that we wait a few weeks and then reconsider what's best to tell them, I think I could live with that. And it will feel better to me if that's a decision we've reached together."

In considering why a particular issue is important to you or your partner, ask yourself these questions: Why is this issue so important? What outcome does either of us really need to have happen in this situation to be content, and what might either of us be willing to let go?

Focus on Possible Solutions

When discussions involve trying to reach decisions about difficult problems, couples often spend more time focusing on what's been wrong and who's to blame than on how to change things. Spending time discussing who's to blame usually is counterproductive to making decisions for at least two reasons. First, people become upset and defensive when they're feeling blamed, and this doesn't encourage them to be cooperative. Second, focusing on the past takes you away from focusing on what you want to do in the future to make things better. The best way to change a conversation that has become focused on deciding who's to blame is to identify this pattern out loud and suggest that, instead, you discuss how to deal with things differently from this point on. Changing the focus to what *you* are willing to change, instead of what you want your partner to change, will also help: "I think we're focusing more right now on who's at fault instead of what each of us could do to make this better in the future. Could we get back to that? How about if I suggest what I think *I* could do to help with this, and then maybe you could give your ideas about what *you* could do."

71

A second tip to remember is that couples often get deadlocked when they focus on only one or two possible solutions, usually with each person trying to gain support for his or her ideas. When you see that happening, try to brainstorm to develop a variety of possible solutions, even if this feels artificial or unsatisfactory. Each of you should try to generate as many possible strategies as you can, even if some ideas seem silly or incomplete. Because the issues that couples in this situation struggle with are often complex and feelings often run strong, we sometimes encourage structuring this brainstorming process by having one partner write down the different solutions each generates so that they're not forgotten in the heat of the moment and can be reconsidered later in the discussion. As solutions are first proposed, you should *not* evaluate them. Instead, work at getting as many different approaches on the table as possible. Often, "suspending critical evaluation" allows new solutions or blends of different solutions to emerge.

Decide on a Solution That Is Agreeable to Both of You

It's likely that no one solution is going to please both you and your partner equally well. That's one reason compromise solutions involving blends of both partners' preferences, or alternating trial periods of both partners' preferences, can sometimes help get a couple unstuck. So look for compromises. Look for ways to incorporate aspects of proposed solutions from each of you. Avoid trying to bully or "guilt" your partner into agreeing with you. Solutions reached under pressure or coercion tend to foster resentment and anger and consequently are likely to fail. Instead, work toward an initial solution that both of you are willing to try, even if you're not sure whether it will work in the long run. Take a risk! Then write down specifically what you've agreed on so there are no questions later.

Decide on a Trial Period

When you write down the solution, agree on a date for it to begin and the length of the initial trial implementation. For certain issues, the decision reached may be "permanent" and won't require a trial period—for example, the decision to end an ongoing affair as a basis for trying to salvage your primary relationship. But agreeing to a trial period often reduces the discomfort of not knowing in advance whether you could live with that decision in the long run.

Bruce and Tina were struggling with how to reorganize their work schedules following Bruce's affair. Tina had always been responsible for getting their children to school, but on some days this got her to work late and she missed critical meetings. She resented that Bruce didn't seem to understand the problems this created for her at work. But when Bruce offered to take over getting the children dressed and fed in the morning and then driving them to school, Tina was anxious that he might not be able to handle this, given the new additional responsibilities of his own at work. They got unstuck when Bruce proposed a 30-day trial period for his taking care of the children in the mornings. If that didn't work, they'd try alternating responsibilities in the morning for the next 30 days. If this still didn't work, they would come back and brainstorm some additional strategies.

So, to sum up: Limit discussions of the past to avoid blame; clarify why an issue is important and brainstorm a variety of solutions; compromise, and then compromise some more; and remember that your decisions can always be renegotiated if they're not successful initially.

Preventing Further Damage

What Should We Do When It Gets Too Heated?

One of the basic principles for talking with each other, identified earlier, is to *prevent further damage*. Despite your best intentions, there may be times when either you or your partner becomes too emotionally upset to engage in discussions about the affair or other relationship issues constructively. You can't express yourself, listen to each other, or reach decisions together effectively when you're so hurt or angry that your feelings take over your thoughts and behaviors. Although such experiences are fairly common among couples struggling to recover from an affair, left unchecked such escalations can create new and even deeper wounds. Sometimes these escalations may even lead to physical altercations. For many couples, learning when and how to take a time-out from destructive interactions is the cornerstone of not making things worse.

What is a *time-out*? Essentially, it's an agreement between you and your partner to take a break from interacting when either one of you feels too angry or too fearful to continue constructively. Try to use time-outs to protect your relationship from harm, not to avoid talking about certain topics simply because they're uncomfortable. Time-outs aren't intended as a way to avoid dealing with difficult issues or as a way to punish your partner for raising difficult issues; instead, they offer a strategy for suspending interactions that seem likely to spiral out of control or cause further damage.

The use of time-outs isn't a complicated concept, but using them constructively can sometimes be difficult. The following guidelines should help. Completing Exercise 3.1 will also help you and your partner to use time-outs to manage discussions that get too heated.

Monitor Your Own Feelings

You and your partner each need to pay attention to your own feelings and recognize when they're getting so intense that you can't interact productively. Common signs might include yelling or getting louder as you speak, not being able to listen to your partner, experiencing excessive muscle tension or lightheadedness, or even feeling an urge to strike out at your partner.

Acknowledge Feelings without Blame

When you feel the need to call a time-out, the goal should be to separate so that you can discuss things together more effectively later. Calling a time-out in an accusatory or blaming way (for example, by saying, "You're getting too emotional and irrational") doesn't help you accomplish this goal. Instead, time-outs work best when you can recognize your own escalating anger and call for a time-out yourself by saying something like "I'm getting too upset to talk more now. I think it might be best if we take a 15-minute time-out before continuing."

Share the Responsibility

Time-outs also work best when couples agree beforehand that *either* partner can call a time-out, including the partner who may be feeling anxious because of the other one's anger. If your partner calls a time-out and expresses concern about your anger, it doesn't necessarily mean that you *are* losing control. What it does mean is that your partner's level of worry about your anger will prevent her from interacting effectively with you until the level of emotions simmers down some. Furthermore, if your partner's emotions feel frightening or destructive to you but your partner doesn't call for a time-out, acknowledge your own discomfort and request a time-out: "I'm concerned that we're just going to get angrier if we continue like this. Let's take a 30-minute time-out and then try again."

Develop a Shared Plan

Time-outs work best if you develop a plan for how you'll handle them in advance. Once you decide to take a time-out, it usually helps if you and your partner go to separate areas. Before you go to separate areas, agree on (1) how long the time-out will last and (2) when and where you'll get back together. This gives both people a sense of what to expect and helps to avoid miscommunications such as "I left because I thought you didn't want to see me again tonight" or "I didn't say that; I just wanted to take a break for a few minutes. You should have known that."

Use the Time-Out Constructively

It's also important to consider what to do and what not to do during a time-out. Going over and over the earlier argument in your mind, for example, is only likely to maintain or increase your anger or other feelings of distress. One way to interrupt your thoughts about the argument is to think of something else instead. Reading a book, watching television, or turning your attention to an unfinished task can distract you from thoughts about the argument. Other techniques for decreasing your distress and becoming calmer include meditation and moderate physical exercise. If going for a walk helps to calm you, be sure you let your partner know where you're going and when you'll be back.

Some people use letter writing as a way of "venting" their feelings or organizing their thoughts. If this works for you, put the letter aside or throw it away when the time-out ends. Letters written in the heat of distress rarely serve constructive purposes when shared later. It's also important not to do anything during the time-out that could potentially be hurtful to you or to others—for example, drinking alcohol or driving when you're upset. Another important use of time-outs is to think about how to interact effectively when you get back together, either thinking about possible solutions to issues you're discussing or trying to clarify your feelings in a nonblaming manner.

Common Hazards

Although there are many ways that time-outs can go wrong, several patterns are particularly common. First, one partner doesn't honor the other person's request to take a time-out. Sometimes partners insist on getting in "the last word." As long as both partners insist on getting in the last word, the end is never reached and the escalation continues. Other times one partner fears that the person leaving won't return and tries to block or restrain the person from leaving. That leads to a physical confrontation that can spiral into aggression. This is why it's so important that a time-out called by either partner be implemented immediately. Also, as mentioned above, it's important not to call a time-out just because an issue feels difficult or uncomfortable.

After the time-out is over, get back together and try discussing the issue again. Don't be surprised if the first couple of times you or your partner are still too upset to discuss things constructively. So if you're still not able to discuss the problem without either one of you getting out of control, take another time-out or suggest an alternative time (for example, the next day) to continue your discussion. Don't try to continue if either one of you is feeling emotionally or physically worn out. Be patient, trust the process, and use time-outs to keep things from getting worse so you can come back and try again at a better time.

Alternative Approaches for Dealing with Intense or "Overheated" Feelings

Writing a Letter as a Way of Expressing Feelings

In our work with couples struggling to recover from an affair, we often suggest letter writing as a way of helping partners express their feelings more effectively. Even those not accustomed to writing about their feelings often see letter writing as an important way of expressing themselves when talking more directly initially fails them.

Letter writing allows you to step back from your feelings to gain a broader perspective and to examine your feelings at a deeper level when you're not immediately confronted with your partner's reactions or challenges. It's often hard to see the big picture, and even harder to *communicate* the big picture, when sharing your feelings elicits hurt, anger, or defensiveness on the part of your partner. Letter writing provides an opportunity to express a more complete picture of what you're experiencing *before* you and your partner get caught up in processing any one particular part of that picture. It provides more opportunity to consider which feelings to emphasize and which ones to omit to get your message across.

Letter writing also increases your opportunity to reflect on your choice of words to express your feelings. How often have you wished you could go back and restate your feelings and express yourself better, only to find that your partner has already latched on to your initial words and that your efforts to "correct" or "amend" your initial message fall on deaf ears? Writing about your feelings in a letter allows you the opportunity to "think before you speak," to consider *how* you want to express yourself, and then to reread what you've written with a "listener's ear" so you can gauge the impact of your message *before* you deliver it. It's important to distinguish between letters written after careful thought and quick notes or e-mails dashed off as a way of venting feelings. The latter rarely contribute to increased understanding and frequently lead to an escalation of angry exchanges—with the additional cost of these being in writing and potentially more enduring.

Similarly, a letter might be easier for your partner to process because he'll be able to take in a more balanced and complete picture before reacting to any one part of your feelings. A letter allows your partner to deal with his initial reaction to your feelings in private and to gain some perspective before responding. In addition, your partner can choose *when* to read your letter, selecting a time when he's less tired, less distressed, and less distracted. Consistent with our earlier guideline to "choose your timing carefully" when *expressing* feelings, letter writing allows the *reader* to select a better time to *receive* the feelings.

How Should I Write the Letter?

The guidelines for letter writing aren't really any different from the guidelines we've already offered for expressing your feelings. Most important is that you try to write a letter that is balanced, focused, and avoids doing further damage. If you're extremely upset or angry, you have two alternatives: (1) wait to write the letter until a later time; or (2) write an initial letter that allows you to "vent" your hurt or frustrations at the time, but destroy the letter afterward. Be sure you distinguish between a letter intended to be shared with your partner, in which you express your feelings in a more selective and softened manner, and one written for the purpose of venting and *not* to be shared with your partner. Letters intended for the purpose of venting that are subsequently "discovered" by your partner can have even more destructive and long-lasting consequences than angry verbal exchanges because they provide a permanent record of your most intense negative feelings.

Begin your letter by identifying your feelings and describing how you're finding it difficult to express those feelings constructively face-to-face. Acknowledge that your feelings stem from your own perspective and that your partner's perspective might be different. Clarify what you're seeking from your partner at this time: understanding of your feelings? clarification of your partner's feelings? reaching a decision together about how to deal with a situation? Keep your letter focused by emphasizing one or two primary feelings and the specific situation giving rise to these feelings. Ask your partner to propose a time and format for responding to your letter—either in a face-to-face discussion or initially in a letter of her own. Exercise 3.2 at the end of this chapter will walk you step-by-step through the process of writing a constructive, thoughtful letter. **Above all, remember that letters aren't intended as a substitute for face-to-face discussions.** Rather, they're a way to express your feelings and thoughts if you think it will be too difficult to talk face-to-face because you'll get upset, your partner won't be able to hear, or an argument is likely to develop.

You can also use letter writing at times when you're not able to *listen* or respond to your partner's feelings in the way you'd like. If you and your partner have tried to talk about an issue several times and it just isn't working, consider using letter writing as a way of working through the impasse. Preparing a letter of response that conveys understanding and empathy is different from writing a letter that focuses on your own thoughts and feelings. In writing a letter of understanding, first acknowledge your own difficulty in listening and responding to your partner's views constructively during the prior discussion, if indeed you did experience difficulty. Avoid using this letter to express your own thoughts and feelings. Instead, as best you can, validate your partner's views by expressing your understanding of how your partner could come to think or feel that way, given his or her perspective. Remember: It's not necessary that you agree with your partner—only that you convey your understanding of the thoughts or feelings your partner has expressed. Then request a time to sit down together and invite your partner to clarify any feelings you're still confused by or to amend or correct any misunderstandings that your letter may include.

If subsequent discussions continue to feel hurtful or to spiral out of control as they did initially, exchange letters again, but this time reverse roles so that you can express your feelings and your partner can communicate his understanding of your perspective. Continue to exchange letters, alternating roles as "speaker" and "listener," until each of you feels more understood and more able to respond with understanding to the other.

What's Next?

After you've completed the following exercises, go on to Chapter 4. There we'll help you develop strategies for dealing with people outside your relationship around issues related to the affair, including setting limits with the outside affair person, deciding what to share with your children, and drawing on support from family and friends while preserving boundaries concerning your privacy.

———————————— Exercises ————————————

EXERCISE 3.1. DESIGNING EFFECTIVE TIME-OUTS

Despite your best intentions, either you or your partner may begin to experience intense feelings during your discussions that make it impossible to continue constructively. If that occurs, it will be helpful if you've already agreed on a specific time-out strategy to implement at such a time.

Write down specific terms for a time-out strategy that you'd like you and your partner to implement if either one of you starts to have feelings that get out of control during your discussion. Your strategy should include:

- *Language for calling the time-out.* For example:

    "I'm starting to feel too angry (or too uncomfortable) to continue this constructively. Let's take a time-out and try again a bit later."

- *Terms of the time-out.* For example:

    "As soon as either one of us calls a time-out, we'll separate and go to different parts of the house for 30 minutes and then return together to the place where we were having the earlier discussion."

- *Terms for deciding to continue.* For example:

  "After the time-out we'll check with each other to see whether the other feels ready to continue the discussion. If not, we'll either (1) extend the time-out for an additional 30 minutes or (2) reschedule for a specific day or time later to try again."

Give your proposal for using time-outs to your partner and invite your partner's reactions or his or her own suggestions for using time-outs constructively. Revise your proposal as necessary, using both your own and your partner's suggestions. What's most important is agreeing on a plan that will effectively suspend discussions that threaten to spiral out of control and that both you and your partner agree to implement.

EXERCISE 3.2. WRITING A LETTER TO YOUR PARTNER

A crucial step in recovering from an affair is understanding the impact of what's happened. You began working toward this understanding with the exercise in Chapter 1 when you examined your initial thoughts, feelings, and behaviors resulting from the affair. The goal of this exercise is to help you communicate these consequences of the affair to your partner. It's important not only that *you* understand what you've been experiencing, but also that *your partner* understand.

The first part of this exercise involves writing a letter to your partner that describes how the affair has affected your thoughts and feelings about your partner, yourself, and your relationship and how these influence how you're acting right now. In the second part of the exercise, your partner writes a letter in response that conveys an understanding of *your* experience as expressed in your letter. In the last part of the exercise, the two of you discuss your respective letters together.

- *If you're working through this book with your partner:* This is the ideal process, and you'll exchange four letters during this exercise. First, the injured partner will write a letter describing the impact of the affair on his or her own thoughts, feelings, and behaviors—and then the participating partner will write a letter in response that summarizes his or her understanding of the injured partner's experience. After an exchange and discussion of these two letters, the participating partner will write a letter describing the impact of the affair for him- or herself. Finally, the injured partner will write a letter conveying his or her understanding of the participating partner's experience.

• *If you're working through this book alone:* You'll still benefit from writing your own letter detailing the impact of the affair on how you think and feel about your partner, yourself, and your relationship. You may consider sharing this letter with your partner even if you don't expect a response, because your own efforts to describe your experience may promote a better understanding between the two of you. Even if you decide not to share your letter, working through this exercise may help you clarify for yourself the impact of the affair.

In preparing your letter, remember to keep your letter balanced, focused, and constructive. In addition, review the guidelines for expressing feelings summarized on pages 58–65. This doesn't mean sugarcoating or minimizing the impact of the affair. But it *does* mean choosing your words carefully and writing about your experience in a way intended to elicit your partner's understanding.

Writing about the Impact of the Affair for Yourself

Write a letter to your partner that describes how the affair has affected your thoughts and feelings about your partner, yourself, and your relationship and how they influence your behavior right now. Try to keep your letter to two to five pages.

Describe how the affair has affected your thoughts, feelings, and behaviors regarding your partner. What feelings are you having toward your partner? For example, how distant or close, anxious or secure, angry or loving do you feel? Use the feeling words listed on page 63. How intense are these thoughts and feelings throughout the day? How much do they fluctuate moment-to-moment? How do these thoughts and feelings influence your interactions with your partner? For example, do they cause you to seek closeness, distance, or both at different times?

Describe how the affair has affected your thoughts, feelings, and behaviors regarding yourself. For example, has the affair caused you to struggle with feelings of unattractiveness, depression, guilt, or shame? How has the affair influenced how you think about yourself? How confused do you feel about your own actions—both prior to and following the affair? How do your thoughts and feelings about yourself influence your interactions with your partner? How do they influence how you're trying to deal with yourself during this time?

Describe how the affair has affected your thoughts, feelings, and behaviors regarding your relationship. How have your thoughts and feelings about your relationship changed as a consequence of the affair? What beliefs have been shattered, and what beliefs have been affirmed? How have your views of your relationship changed, in either positive or negative ways? Given what's happened, how sure are you about what you wish for your relationship in the long term? In what ways do these thoughts and feelings influence your ability or motivation to work on your relationship?

When you've finished writing your letter, put it aside for a day. Then come back and read through it, asking yourself the following questions:

- *Is your letter balanced?* Does the language accurately convey both the depth and complexity of thoughts and feelings? Does the letter reflect any feelings of hope as well as despair? Any wishes for closeness in addition to impulses to retreat?
- *Is your letter complete?* Have you expressed both thoughts and feelings—as well as their influence on your actions—regarding the affair's impact on your experience of your partner, yourself, and your relationship?
- *Is your letter constructive?* Does it express your thoughts and feelings in a way that your partner will be able to hear?

If you've answered no to any of these questions, wait another day or two and try revising your letter to communicate more effectively the impact of the affair for you. After you're confident that your letter accurately conveys your experience in each of the three areas we've outlined—and does so in a manner intended to elicit your partner's understanding as constructively as possible—give the letter to your partner and allow him or her the opportunity to read through it at a separate time and place.

Writing about the Impact of the Affair for Your Partner

Write a letter to your partner that describes how the affair has affected your partner's thoughts and feelings about you, about him- or herself, and about your relationship. This isn't a time to write about *your own* experience. Rather, it's your opportunity to convey how well you truly understand *your partner's* experience.

Begin your letter by expressing your appreciation for your partner's willingness to share his or her thoughts and feelings and how they're influencing your partner's interactions with you. Try to summarize the major themes or primary feelings contained in your partner's letter. Specifically, how has the affair affected your partner's thoughts and feelings about you, about him- or herself, and about your relationship? Try to use your own words to describe *your partner's* experience as a way of conveying your understanding.

Do the best you can to validate your partner's views by expressing your understanding of how your partner could come to think or feel that way, given his or her own perspective. Remember: It's not necessary that you agree with your partner—only that you convey your understanding of the thoughts or feelings that he or she has expressed.

When you've finished writing your letter, put it aside for a day. Then come back and read through it, asking yourself the following questions:

- *Have you focused on summarizing your partner's experience rather than describing your own?*
- *Have you acknowledged the full range of thoughts and feelings conveyed in your partner's letter?* Have you recognized both positive and negative feelings, if these were expressed? Have you covered each of the areas addressed by your partner—specifically, the impact of the affair on your partner's experience of you, him- or herself, and your relationship?
- *Have you affirmed your partner's perspective?* That is, have you conveyed your own understanding of how your partner could come to think and feel this way, given your partner's particular viewpoint?

After you're confident that your letter conveys your best understanding of your partner's experience, give the letter to your partner and allow him or her the opportunity to read through it at a separate time and place.

Discussing Your Letters

Once both letters have been exchanged, agree on a time to sit down and discuss them. Begin with the first partner's letter expressing the impact of the affair on him- or herself; then proceed to the other partner's letter of understanding. Try to clarify any feelings that are still confusing to either of you. If your discussion begins to feel destructive or spirals out of control, take a time-out using the guidelines discussed earlier in this chapter. After you've exchanged and discussed this first set of letters, consider repeating this exercise with the roles of "speaker" and "listener" reversed.

4

>>>————————————————————————————

How Do We Deal
with Others?

Ellen couldn't get Kate out of her mind. Rob insisted that their affair was over, that he avoided contact with Kate and made sure they were never alone together at the office. That wasn't enough for Ellen. Rob finally felt pushed to request a move to a different work team. Now Rob saw Kate only for a brief moment every few weeks, at a meeting on her floor. Ellen had hoped this arrangement would make her comfortable, but even if she learned to trust Rob again, she would never trust Kate. The only solution in Ellen's mind was for Rob to leave the company. Rob initially resisted, but finally gave in to what he viewed as Ellen's ultimatum and resigned.

A slow economy made it hard for Rob to find another job with equal pay or status, so he took a less prestigious job with a significant pay cut. He felt like a failure professionally and resented Ellen for "forcing" him to change jobs as a way of "punishing" him for the affair. So he felt fully justified in pushing her to return to work to make up for his pay cut. He didn't like having to put their daughter in day care after he and Ellen had initially agreed that Ellen would stay home during her preschool years. "That's life," he told himself. Ellen's anger toward Rob grew day by day. Not only had he betrayed her as a husband, but now he had forced her to betray their daughter as well. Rob's and Ellen's bitterness toward each other festered. After two years, they concluded there was little between them to salvage and ended their marriage in a bitter divorce.

How should you deal with your partner's interactions with the outside affair person? Should you and your partner confront the person together? Should you trust your partner to end it on his own? Should you insist on no further contact, even if that means switching jobs?

Your partner will need to think about how he feels about these issues too. If he and the person he had the affair with are likely to cross paths, is he willing to change jobs, or even move to a new community, to avoid these encounters? Should he do so?

Did Ellen and Rob make a good decision? Could their marriage have been saved if they had come up with another way to limit Rob's contact with Kate to make Ellen feel secure? Ellen had consulted her mother, who agreed that Rob's resigning was the only chance Ellen had to save her marriage. Was Ellen right to bring in her mother?

Although an affair affects you and your partner most directly, it may have an impact on your other relationships too. Each of you now must decide whom to tell about the affair—and what to tell. How will you respond if others ask you about what's happening? What do you want, if anything, from them? Although there are no absolute answers to most of these questions, some general principles can guide you in making such decisions.

How Do We Decide Whom to Tell about the Affair?

You may have to tell some people about the affair—your boss needs to know why you can't work with a colleague any longer, or your child's day care worker needs to understand why your child is anxious these days. Or you may feel you should tell some people, such as when your closest friend might feel hurt by the realization that you're keeping something important to yourself. And if you need help or support—say, from a sibling whom you can count on to be there for you—you'll have to explain why. The important factor in deciding whom to tell is *to be clear and honest with yourself about why you're talking to that person.*

This means exploring *all* the motives you might have, not just the "good" ones. You might believe your children deserve to know what's happened because it affects them. But is there a part of you that wants to punish your partner or get your children on your side? Are you pushing your partner to tell the boss "for the welfare of the company," when your secret hope is that the outside person will be fired? Are you planning on sending an anonymous letter to the outside person's partner because it's the "right thing" to let her know she needs to be evaluated for sexually transmitted diseases, when what you really want is to see their marriage in a shambles just like yours? It's not hard to come up with "good" reasons for telling someone about the affair when there are unrecognized motives that may be less virtuous. Wanting to get back at your partner or the outside person is understandable and can feel good in the moment. Acting on that desire, however, often has negative long-term consequences.

Once you know for sure why you want to tell someone about the affair, also think carefully about whether this person is appropriate to turn to for this purpose. For example, should you turn to your children for emotional support while going through this crisis, or are there others who can provide such support without placing your children in an adult's role? (In the section beginning on page 99, we discuss in detail what to tell the children and how to interact with them.) Is it appropriate to ask a couple that you two see together to support you individually or take sides against your partner? Suppose you and your partner eventually decide to remain together. If you turned to a family member for advice on getting through this difficult time, might that person forever resent your partner for hurting you? Should you contact a clergyperson or a mental health professional instead? *Identifying what you need and finding an appropriate person to meet that need is critical to the recovery process.*

How Do We Deal with the Outside Affair Person?

Following an affair, you need to determine whether you can restore a sense of trust and control in your life, and the person your partner had the affair with can be a major obstacle to recovery. Whether the affair has ended or not, the outside person is a major part of the trauma you've experienced and may be an ongoing threat.

The most important issue to address regarding the outside person is how to set boundaries around your relationship and protect it from further intrusion. Without appropriate boundaries, you won't be able to create the sense of safety that will help you move forward as a couple. Continued interactions between your partner and the outside person can feel threatening, may increase the likelihood that the affair will rekindle, and can lead to ongoing emotional turmoil for everyone. But limiting or eliminating contact can be difficult—because the participating partner and the other person work together, because the outside person may pursue continued contact even though the affair is over, or because the affair hasn't ended yet.

>>> **You can overcome these obstacles by keeping the following guidelines in mind:**
- **Understand that, typically, the stronger and firmer the boundaries, the better for your relationship.**
- **Don't make agreements you can't keep or will resent.**
- **Remember that discussing these boundaries is a process that takes time, and your decisions may change as time passes.**

You and your partner need to have a series of conversations in which you clarify the current status of the relationship with the outside person, express how each of you feels about continued interaction and whether the outside person is willing to let go, and decide on what boundaries to set. *These discussions and negotiations can include some of the most difficult initial issues that couples address when an affair becomes known.* The injured person will find it painful even to consider possible further contact with the outside person, and the participating partner will have to deal with feeling guilt, shame, anger, or sadness without being permitted to have or express those feelings.

Because these discussions can be so upsetting, some couples avoid them. Some participating partners believe that if the affair is over they don't need to discuss the outside person. In our experience, however, this kind of avoidance generally doesn't work. *The outside person's continued presence is a critical threat, and you two need to discuss what boundaries to set.*

What Boundaries Should We Set If the Affair Has Ended?

Derek's affair with Renee was supposed to end two months ago, but she was so devastated by the idea of losing him that Derek reluc-

tantly agreed that they could be "just friends." Renee took this as a sign that Derek didn't really want to break it off after all. But when he didn't return her advances when they met, she was enraged and started calling Derek's home every night. When Derek's wife answered the phone, Renee taunted Shelley with details of their rendezvous. Everything the couple had done to try to save their marriage fell apart in the constant arguments over how to end Renee's persistent intrusions. Shelley was bitter and angry about the turmoil that Derek had brought into their lives.

Set Clear, Strong Boundaries Following the Affair

The stronger and firmer the boundaries and the less interaction with the outside person, the better. *Trying to remain friends with someone after an affair becomes known rarely works; at least one of the three people in this triangle is likely to find the arrangement unacceptable.* We said earlier that these boundaries are critical to restoring the sense of security shattered by the affair. Your partner's continued interactions with the outside person will just keep reopening those old wounds, making it seem as if the threat will never go away. Doing the work you need to do to explore rebuilding your relationship is going to make you feel vulnerable to your partner in the first days and weeks following an affair, and unless you have some way of feeling safe, this work will feel too risky to undertake.

Continued interaction doesn't serve the participating partner well either when the goal is to end the affair and move on. Contact with the outside person can rekindle positive feelings, create confusion over important relationship decisions, and distract the participating partner with worry about how these meetings could be misinterpreted or guilt over hiding the fact that they're occurring in the first place. And, as with Renee, continuing any kind of relationship can delude the outside person into believing that the participating partner really doesn't want to end the affair.

The bottom line is this: Continued interactions with the outside person usually keep someone or everyone in continued turmoil.

You and your partner will need to establish clear expectations regarding any future contact—how an interaction might come about and how to address it. You'll need to decide whether *any type of communication* is acceptable, as well as whether *any setting for interaction* is acceptable. Exercise 4.1 will help you do this. For example, is a telephone conversation okay, but not face-to-face contact? Is e-mail correspondence acceptable? Many people have a very clear answer to all of these questions: "No, nothing is acceptable." However, at times this response is unrealistic, at least right away. If, for example, your partner and the outside person work together and the affair has just become known, it might be unrealistic to say, "Never speak to that person again about anything." That's why the *setting for interactions* needs to be considered. Even if the participating and outside person work and typically travel together, you as a couple may decide that for now group interaction in a business meeting is acceptable but travel and one-on-one meetings are not. Similarly, group business lunches might seem okay, but one-on-one business dinners might not.

Implied in these examples is a third factor: the *topic or focus* of what is discussed during the interactions. Many couples set a boundary that there's to be no discussion of personal relationships or feelings with the outside person, but necessary communications about work or about ending the relationship are acceptable for a short time. For example, business interactions may be allowed in some circumstances, or telephone calls to end the relationship or to tell the outside person to have no further contact of any type might be needed. We know that disclosure of personal feelings is one of the major ways that people develop an intimate relationship. Therefore, conversations between the participating partner and outside person about how much they care about each other, how much they miss each other, and what sense of loss they're experiencing create a high-risk situation. Self-disclosure leads to more self-disclosure, which then leads to greater feelings of intimacy.

At times, some interaction with the outside person may be needed to establish the ground rules about boundaries. As a couple, you should decide on the message and mode of delivery, such as an e-mail message signed by you as a couple. After Paco told Elena about his affair, they decided to write an e-mail message together, which Paco then sent:

> *"I've told my wife, Elena, about our affair and that I've decided to end it. We're going to work on our marriage. I know that this decision will be painful for you; it is for all of us. But I've given it a lot of thought, and that is what I'm going to do. I'm asking you not to call or come to see me; just send me a reply saying you've received this message. In a couple of days, I'll contact you, and I hope we can meet in some*

public setting to say good-bye. After that meeting, I want to ask that we have no further contact of any sort; I need to move on with my life and work on my marriage. I truly am sorry for all the pain I have caused all of us. Paco."

Make Realistic Agreements

Together, you're attempting to create a relationship built on honesty, trust, and safety. Promising to limit interactions with the outside person and then not doing so undermines these goals. Therefore, it's important to *agree only to what you know you can do*, even if that means renegotiating as time passes. Sometimes it makes sense to agree to take it a day at a time, not to renegotiate limits every single day but to be alert to the need to do so as it arises.

> *Although Jeff wanted Heather to end all contact with Kurt, Heather felt too ambivalent about her marriage with Jeff to end the affair immediately. She knew she couldn't in truth agree to no contact. She summoned up her nerve to express these feelings to Jeff. After some painful negotiation, they agreed she could communicate with Kurt via e-mail, but she needed to let Jeff know what she was saying. They also agreed that she would maintain this kind of contact only for a limited time while she was working with an individual therapist on deciding what she wanted to do. At the end of the trial period, they would reassess the situation and Heather would have to make a decision.*

View Setting Limits as an Ongoing Process

You don't know how you'll react over time to the limits you've set. So use the decision-making guidelines in Chapter 3 to make the best decision you can and set a trial period. If you find at the end of the trial period the decision isn't working, find a new solution together.

Viewing the limit setting as an ongoing process also means recognizing how relationships work and change over time. This consideration is particularly important if the affair hasn't yet ended. If you discovered your partner's ongoing affair, your first instinct may have been to demand that your partner promise to cease all forms of interaction with the other person from that moment forward. Feeling frightened and having received an ultimatum, your partner might have agreed, only to fail to keep the agreement. Rarely will someone instantly end a meaningful relationship without any further contact with the other person. For better or worse, relationships usually just don't end that way. Therefore, couples should discuss what's realistic, what the participating partner needs to do to end the affair, and how to structure any future interactions that do occur.

At the same time, however, a participating partner shouldn't use these recommendations as an excuse to continue an affair or to take advantage of an injured partner. If you've decided to end an affair, end it as quickly and definitely as possible. Not all injured partners behave angrily and give ultimatums. Some are depressed or worried about losing a partner and are hesitant to set limits. Both partners need to take responsibility for setting and respecting limits. If you're the participating partner, don't focus on trying to get by with or talk your partner into as much as you can. Your focus needs to be on repairing your relationship and attending to your partner. *Take responsibility for establishing limits, and arrange your life so you can abide by them.* Our guidelines regarding types of communication, settings for interacting with the outside person, and the content of conversations aren't intended merely to satisfy or placate your partner. They're designed to help you, the participating partner, follow through on agreements. There may be moments when your warm feelings for the outside person return. If so, having private conversations and discussing personal feelings dramatically increase the risk for resuming the affair. Establishing and respecting strong, consistent boundaries can help you get through difficult times.

When the Affair Has Ended

- Make limits on any future contact very clear.
- Be specific about how the participating partner is supposed to tell the injured partner when those limits have been violated.
- Agree on a plan for responding if the outside person initiates contact.
- If necessary, tell the outside person again that the affair has ended.
- If circumstances require some continued contact (such as at work), be clear about limits on the setting and focus for these interactions.

How Do We Respond If the Outside Person Makes Contact?

Even when an affair has ended and your partner faithfully honors the limits set for interacting with the outside person, you need to decide together what to do if there's a chance meeting or one initiated by the outside person. *The most important principle is for the participating partner to inform the injured partner of any such interactions and disclose what happened—however the meeting came about.*

"The last thing in the world I want to do is tell Janice that Gwen e-mailed me," Tim protested. "We're doing better, so why rock the boat by bringing that up? I didn't respond to the e-mail, so why not let sleeping dogs lie?" Tim's reaction is understandable, but there are important reasons to tell his wife about the e-mail message. First, failing to disclose it reflects continued deceit and secrecy and works against Tim's pledge to rebuild a truthful relationship with Janice, whether she finds out or not. And if Janice does learn about the contact, the attempts at rebuilding trust are damaged even more deeply. Finally, there's probably nothing Tim can do that will be more powerful to rebuild trust than to share this information. Because Janice is most worried about whether Tim will renew his affair, if he consistently tells her when Gwen contacts him, Janice can begin to trust Tim and feel that they're working together as a team. Disclosing interactions with the outsider can be painful in the short run, but usually rebuilds trust in the long run. Therefore, our advice here is simple and direct: *If you want to rebuild a trusting relationship with your partner, disclose interactions with the outside person, no matter how trivial these interactions may seem.*

The flip side of this advice involves the injured partner's response to receiving such information. Learning that your partner and the outside person have had some kind of contact almost always feels threatening and painful. A natural impulse is to lash out at your partner. But doing so, particularly when the contact was initiated by the outside person and beyond your partner's control, punishes rather than strengthens your partner's efforts to risk difficult feelings for the sake of rebuilding trust. As an injured partner, it's critical for you to distinguish between exchanges initiated by your partner and those resulting from intrusions by the outside person. If the interaction results from behaviors of the outside person, it's still okay to express feelings of anxiety, hurt, or anger, but be sure also to let your partner know that you're not holding him responsible for the *current* exchange. In other words, be sure to distinguish between the hurt or anger you have from the affair itself and your feelings about the recent interaction with the outside person that your partner is describing to you now.

Besides being scrupulously honest about interactions that occur, you need to resolve to take whatever steps are necessary to stop the outside person from unwanted intrusions into your relationship. Partners may decide to act together—for example, by writing and signing a letter from both partners, sending a joint e-mail message, making a joint telephone call, or asking to meet together with the person in a public setting. Donna and Sam decided to make a joint telephone call to Gary the morning before the couple left together on vacation. Although Donna had broken off her affair with Gary months earlier, Gary continued to send e-mails to Donna, professing how much he missed her. Although some couples may not choose to start a vacation this way, for Donna and Sam it was a symbolic way of bringing closure before beginning their vacation together. They told Gary they were both on the line, although Donna did all the talking for them. This voice of unity was important as they told Gary that he and Donna could have no further contact, ever.

When the Outside Person Doesn't Want to Let Go

- Discuss other ways to get the message across to the outside person that the affair is over.
- Examine possible "mixed messages" and make sure they're not sent anymore.
- When these strategies fail, seek assistance in limiting contact—from supervisors if the affair arose at work or through legal action if necessary.
- In extreme circumstances, consider moving to another community.

Unfortunately, at times such messages fall on deaf ears. An outside person who refuses to let go may attempt to destroy the marriage, seduce the partner, threaten to kill herself, or threaten the injured partner or a member of her family. Take such threats seriously, and consider getting outside assistance. We've worked with couples who've hired a lawyer to draft a letter threatening legal action if the outside person didn't stop harassing them. Some couples contact the police to issue a restraining order. Many states also have antistalking laws intended to prevent persistent, unwanted intrusions when the recipient has told the stalker to stop and the recipient feels physically unsafe. Finally, if all these measures have failed, if the outside person is a danger to you or others, or if the outside person is destroying your relationship, you can consider the last resort of moving to a different community. We know of couples who have moved across the country to get away from someone who simply would not give up on an affair. Strategies for how to respond when the outside person doesn't want to let go are listed in the box on the facing page.

What Boundaries Should We Set If the Affair Is Still Going On?

If you're in the dreadful position of having found out about your partner's ongoing affair, and your partner doesn't realize you know, confronting your partner about the affair and deciding what to do is the first critical step. Although there are few absolutes in dealing with affairs, our experience with scores of couples has shown that colluding with your partner to allow an affair to continue in the hope that it will end on its own is unlikely to work. If you've already confronted your partner, and he has refused to end the affair at the present time, it's probably because he's proposing an ongoing "open" marriage or relationship or he's uncertain whether to continue your relationship or the relationship with the outside person. In the first situation, think carefully before you agree to a so-called open marriage. Most people consider accepting such an arrangement out of fear of losing their marriages, or because they've become convinced that their attitudes toward sexual exclusivity are too conservative, old-fashioned, or prudish. Although you or your partner may know of unusual or nontraditional arrangements that appear to work for some couples, in our experience open marriages are rarely successful in the long term in our society. Typically, either one person's need for an emotionally intimate relationship doesn't allow for sharing the partner with someone else, or the only way the marriage can remain open is to limit emotional intimacy altogether, making for a relationship that eventually becomes distant and unsatisfying.

More likely if your partner refuses to end an affair, it's because your partner finds that relationship intensely rewarding. Sometimes a person doesn't actually want to leave his or her marriage for the other person, but the relationship with the outsider is so gratifying in some ways that the person doesn't want to end it until absolutely necessary. If this is the case in your relationship, we recommend that you do the following: *Make it necessary*. Specifically, clearly state your unwillingness to accept an ongoing affair in the long run and be adamant that your partner work toward difficult decisions about how to resolve this. Giving up the gratification of a novel sexual relationship or the emotional intimacy of a relationship with few responsibilities is hard for many people. In such cases, set firm limits on your partner, but don't give premature ultimatums or ones that can't be honored.

Mark explained his affair by saying he wasn't particularly unhappy with his marriage to Fran but really did want the opportunity to be with other women. He was middle-aged, overcome with responsibilities, and felt the need to be free to do what he wanted. They tried an "open" marriage, but it drove Fran "crazy." Fran agreed to wait two months, and at the end of that time either the affair had to be over or their marriage would be. At the end of that time Mark ended the affair, and he and Fran continued to work on their marriage in couple therapy.

Of course, not every situation has this outcome. In setting limits, injured partners can sometimes push the participating partner further into the affair. Keith refused to even speak with Sarah for several weeks after learning of her affair, hoping this would force her to end it; instead, it convinced Sarah that she and Keith would never be able to discuss what had gone wrong in their marriage, and within a few months she ended both the affair and her marriage. In deciding on what limits to set, you have to decide for yourself whether you're prepared to take this risk. The important point is not to allow yourself to contribute to an ongoing situation that you can't tolerate or that is destructive to either of you.

If your partner is undecided about whether to continue the affair versus ending it to preserve your own relationship, you already know how distressing this is. You may feel naive for allowing your partner to continue the other relationship. If you've told your friends, they may tell you that you're crazy to allow it, or they may recommend a private detective to get a good divorce settlement or suggest similar strategies to pursue. At the same time, you may feel reluctant to force the issue because your partner might choose the other person. You may realize that comparing your current relationship to an affair with its novelty, thrill of secrecy, and few daily demands can place your own relationship at a disadvantage. So, what should you do if your partner seems unwilling to end an affair because of ambivalence regarding long-term intentions?

No single answer to this question works equally well for everyone. We urge you to ignore anyone who offers a definitive answer, whether that person is a family member, friend, professional, or author of another self-help book. It's important to understand the risks of pursuing any option and to be willing to live with the potential consequences. What are the major risks of allowing a partner to continue an affair in order to have time to decide what to do? The primary risk is that some participating partners will settle into long-term or semipermanent indecision. We've worked with couples who had been in this state of indecision for five years or longer before seeking professional assistance. They hadn't agreed to an open marriage; rather, they simply hadn't decided what to do. Why? Because reaching a decision in one direction or the other meant giving up something enjoyable or risking something valuable. Often the participating partner doesn't want to end either the marriage or the affair; both feel important, and ending either one creates significant loss. Therefore, some participating partners simply don't decide between the two relationships; in other words, they decide *not* to decide.

Similarly, for a variety of reasons the injured partner often is reluctant to force the issue of the partner's affair. If you're the injured person, you may truly love your partner; you've built a life and a family together, and you don't want to end this phase of your life. You may endure your participating partner's indecision because you fear the answer that might be given if you force the issue. You may believe you can't survive without your partner, emotionally or otherwise. Or you may worry about your children's welfare and be willing to endure your own personal pain to keep your family intact. Perhaps economic factors make it difficult for you to challenge your partner's affair; for women in particular, divorce often leads to economic hardship.

What are the possible benefits of allowing an affair to continue? On a short-term basis, it permits the couple to delay painful decisions about the future. In some cases, affairs run their course, they eventually end, and the husband and wife continue with their marriage. Although there's limited research on this issue, it appears that only a small fraction of people having affairs—possibly as low as 10%—actually divorce their partners and then marry the outside person. In other words, the prevailing image of participating partners "running off with" the outsider doesn't hold up in most cases. (The limited research also suggests that most marriages born out of an affair end in divorce.) Sometimes it may be reasonable to delay forcing a decision, particularly if the couple is actively engaged in confronting the affair and discussing what steps to take to move forward.

Alternatively, what are the benefits and risks of forcing a decision regarding an ongoing affair? For some injured partners forcing the issue is a way of regaining a sense of control when life has felt very much out of control. It's a way of affirming your own worth and saying, "I deserve better than this. I won't let you treat me or our relationship this way." Many people feel emotionally abused when a partner continues an affair, and forcing a decision is a way of ending the mistreatment. If the couple's relationship survives, then the injured partner has defined what will be tolerated in the future. Moreover, requiring a decision about the outside relationship ends the immediate nightmare; the injured partner may be right in believing that he just can't go on this way any longer.

The major risk in pushing for a decision is that the participating partner may decide to end the marriage when the injured partner still wants very much to continue it. If your relationship with your partner feels particularly bad, and your partner's affair seems particularly important or rewarding, your partner may indeed end your relationship prematurely, even declaring that your forcing the issue caused this outcome. In these circumstances, forcing the issue too early may deprive the two of you of an opportunity to examine your relationship and begin the difficult work of restoring it.

If it appears, for whatever reasons, that a partner's affair is going to continue for some time, it's still important to discuss what types of boundaries to set regarding the outside person. An ongoing affair doesn't necessarily mean it's okay for the partner to come and go or behave as she pleases. For example, you might negotiate whether phone calls to or from the outside person are to be allowed at your home. If you're going to be away, you might want an agreement about whether the outside person is ever to come to your home. If you have children, you may decide together about whether the children are to have any knowledge of or contact with the outside person. (We'll discuss children in more detail in the next section of this chapter.) Or you might want to reach an agreement about whether the partner and outside person are to appear together in public or remain in private settings only.

Some couples separate while an affair is ongoing, and if you do, these conversations are still important. It's important to make short-term agreements while you decide together about the future of your relationship. For example, you may need to decide how to handle your finances, how to interact either separately or together around your children's activities, whether to continue with family trips, and so on. How long are you willing to live with any interim agreement? Be sure both you and your partner understand that you'll likely need to renegotiate some of these agreements. Sometimes injured partners find that certain agreements are simply too distressing to continue. After a trial period, you may need to rework unacceptable agreements or push for a decision about the affair.

We know you may be facing a painful dilemma if your partner refuses to end an affair but is also asking not to end your relationship. You and your partner have to live with the consequences of your decisions, so be very careful as you consider any well-intended advice from others. It can be just as reasonable to decide to stay for now as to push for a decision. *Take the time you need; making a major life decision when you're upset, tired, or worn down can be risky.* At these times many people find that a professional trained to help with difficult life decisions gives them a useful outside perspective.

When the Affair Is Still Going On

- Distinguish between intermediate- and long-term goals. Be realistic about what to expect in the short term.
- Agree on a time frame for the participating partner to reach a decision regarding the affair.
- Define the limits, if any, on the nature of continued contact.
- Develop specific guidelines for communicating with each other about either partner's contact with the outside person.
- Be clear about next steps to pursue once the participating partner decides to end the affair or if either partner decides to end the marriage.

What Do We Tell the Children and How Do We Interact with Them?

Margaret was devastated by Liam's affair. She had never thought it possible that he would do this to her and their children, and she was determined that he wouldn't get away with it. She told both of their teenage daughters what their father had done and waited to see their outrage. She wasn't prepared for the depth of their hurt and confusion. Years later, Margaret's oldest daughter confessed that knowing about her father's affair still haunted her in her own romantic relationships, and she described how much she had hated being caught between him and her mother.

If you have children and one of you is having an affair, you've probably been thinking about this important question: "What do we tell the children?" Children of most ages are aware when there's heightened distress. You and your partner may argue more often or intensely; you might spend less time together; or either one of you may show various signs of more acute anxiety or sadness. It seems important to say or do something, but what? First, be guided by this general principle: *In deciding what to say and do, make your children's well-being your top concern.* Beyond that, make the guidelines in the box below your mantra; refer to them often as a reminder after reading the explanations that follow. Exercise 4.2 will also help you reach decisions about how to interact with your children about the affair.

Guidelines for Dealing with Children

- Help your children maintain caring and loving relationships with both parents.
- Say only what is necessary.
- Adjust what you say to your children's ages and levels of development.
- Minimize the disruption of your children's lives.
- Avoid allowing your children to become your parents and take care of you during this crisis.

Help Your Children Maintain Caring and Loving Relationships with Both Parents

When the relationship between you and your partner is disrupted, your children need the safety and security of strong relationships with both parents. You may want a chance to explain your side of the story so as not to be blamed for what's happening in the marriage. As the injured partner, you may feel your partner doesn't deserve your children's love and affection. When such thoughts cross your mind, always come back to principle number one: If it's not in your children's best interest, it's not the right choice. And it's definitely not in their best interest to experience such a loss. A great deal of research indicates that children can endure a wide variety of their parents' marital conflicts, including divorce, if they can maintain loving relationships with both parents and not have to choose sides between them. At times, you may need to "bite your tongue" and refrain from saying what you would like to say to your children about your partner. We don't advocate that you lie to your children; however, you need to consider carefully what to share and what to keep to yourself. A key factor to consider in what to disclose about the affair is how it will impact your children's relationships with both parents.

Say Only What Is Necessary

The central question for most parents is whether to tell the children explicitly that one partner has had or is having an affair. Some experts argue that children should *always* be told about an affair, using language appropriate to their age. Children will always find out anyway, certain writers claim, so they should be told by their parents. Others claim children should be informed of an affair because they are a central part of the family. Actually, there's no evidence that children inevitably find out about their parents' extramarital affairs, so be cautious in accepting this logic. If many people know about the affair, including your children's friends or their parents, and your children are likely to learn about it, you may want to tell them yourselves so that you have some control over what they hear and how they hear it. As to whether the children *should* know everything that goes on in their family, the competing philosophy that the intimate details of an adult couple's lives are private and aren't necessarily to be shared with children is equally valid. This is your call.

It is important to talk with children, however, when there's significant distress in your relationship. They're likely to experience that *something* is wrong but may be confused without additional information. Consequently, it's important to acknowledge that Mom and Dad aren't getting along and are unhappy with each other right now. It also can be helpful for children to know what will change and what will remain the same. For example, you may want to let them know that you might not be doing as many things together as a family but will continue to live together.

In many instances there's no clear reason why the children need to know about an affair unless it's likely to become public knowledge. Just as you'd be unlikely to tell the children about difficulties in your sexual relationship, you don't necessarily need to tell them about the *specific basis* of other relationship problems. What your children need help in understanding is the general magnitude of their parents' conflicts and their likely effects—that is, what's likely to change or remain the same in their own lives. *Remember that the **most** important information your children need is that both parents still love them very much.*

Adjust What You Say to Your Children's Age and Level of Development

Whatever you say to your children, use language that they can comprehend based on their age and level of development. For example, if you're speaking to a seven-year-old, you'd be unlikely to say, "Your father's having an extramarital affair with Mrs. Jones." Instead, if you're going to raise the issue of an affair with your seven-year-old, you might say, "Your dad isn't sure he wants to continue being married to me. He's found someone else that he cares about a lot, so let me tell you what's going to happen."

Not only must you decide *what* to tell your children, but you also have to decide *how* to tell them. Although there are no absolute rules that fit all situations, it is generally true that if you're telling your children about your relationship difficulties, it may be beneficial if you and your partner talk with them together. Conversely, if your children are far apart in age, you may want to talk with each child separately so that you can adjust what you say to the level of development of each. However, in many cases, it works best to gather the family together and tell everyone at once. Having both parents present to talk to the children can prevent either one of you from presenting the situation in a blaming way. It also keeps your discussion on a family level, emphasizing that you, the parents, are having difficulty and that you'll approach the problem together. Children often have questions, and if both parents are present, it's easier to provide answers. Saying, "Talk to your father [or mother] about that" can sound implicitly blaming or can force your child to wait to have important questions answered. Finally, if you and your partner each present your own version of the relationship struggles separately, the inevitable differences or inconsistencies in your accounts will lead to confusion for your children or possibly their feeling caught in the middle between you.

Despite these considerations, some couples decide to have each parent talk with the children separately. Usually this option is chosen when the two partners are so angry with each other that they can't guarantee they can avoid a confrontation in front of the children. Likewise, some partners are fairly certain that they'll become upset, cry, or be unable to get through a discussion with the children if the other partner is present.

In such cases, either go ahead and talk to the children separately or wait until you're able to interact with each other less negatively, if that seems possible in the foreseeable future. If you decide to talk to your children separately, make sure you've discussed what each of you will say, how you'll handle certain issues that might come up, and how you'll try to avoid blaming each other or putting your children in the middle of your own struggles.

Minimize the Disruption to Your Children's Lives

When you talk to your children about your relationship problems, they may become worried and anxious or sad and depressed. Some get into trouble with arguments, fights, or poor school performance; and others, at least outwardly, seem almost indifferent to the family crisis. Regardless of how your children respond, recognize that the upcoming months may be very difficult for them. Their lives may feel unpredictable and beyond their control. As you've experienced yourself, loss of control and unpredictability are usually frightening. *Do whatever you can to maintain your children's typical daily routine.*

Meanwhile, don't deny the difficulties your family is experiencing. Be sure to talk with your children as needed about any significant changes, particularly changes in residence, as well as both parents' ongoing participation in meals, school activities, church, or family vacations. Other than consequences of your relationship difficulties that directly influence them, keep the details to yourselves, although you might consider telling the children if you and your partner are seeking professional help in working on your relationship.

Avoid Allowing Your Children to Become Your Parents and Take Care of You During this Crisis

During this difficult time you may need lots of support, both emotional and practical. Emotional support usually involves having someone listen to your concerns, offer understanding, and care for you emotionally. Although it's certainly appropriate for your children to behave in ways that reflect care and concern for you, it's also important that they remain in their proper roles. Your children shouldn't be the ones you turn to for support, understanding, empathy, or advice while you discuss what's happening in your marriage, whether your children are still young or even if they're grown. *Turning to your children for emotional support often forces them to choose between their two parents, an unfair choice for you to impose at any age.*

Aside from emotional support, when people are under a lot of stress they often need extra practical support or help with various tasks. You may find that you have less energy than usual. If you and your partner are living apart, there may simply be more to do; alternatively, if you and your partner are still living together, you may be reluctant to ask your partner to do certain things because your relationship feels so chaotic. Although it might be appropriate to ask children to help out more during these difficult times, be careful not to overdo it. Don't ask a child to become "the man (or woman) of the house" because your partner is emotionally or physically absent. Sometimes a child who is highly conscientious and responsible begins to behave more like a parent during these difficult times, particularly if you or your partner is struggling. This reversal of roles is almost always detrimental to the child, either short term or long term. Having children who help out can be wonderful, but make certain that the children continue to be children, functioning in a way that's appropriate for their age and level of individual development.

What Do We Tell Family Members and Friends?

In a fit of rage, Luis told his family about Ramona's affair. As he had hoped, his family rallied around him in support and in anger at her betrayal. However, in the following weeks Luis decided that he really loved Ramona and didn't want to end their marriage. As they both worked to rebuild their relationship, his family's support turned to anger at Luis. They couldn't understand how he could take her back, labeling him weak and foolish. Ramona was furious at their treatment of both her and Luis, and they both ended up feeling isolated from his family.

You're likely to tell family members or friends about an affair for either of two reasons: (1) You think they should know or have the right to know, or (2) you want or need something from them, probably some type of support. Everyone has a different set of family and friend relationships, so you need to decide who should know about your current difficulties and exactly what they should know. You may decide to tell family members and friends that you're having difficulties, but not share with them that one of you has had an extramarital affair. In other cases, you may have a close and trusting relationship with a family member or friend whose specific assistance or advice regarding the affair could be quite valuable. The guidelines summarized in the box below are discussed more thoroughly on the next few pages. Exercise 4.3 will also help you reach decisions about talking with others about the affair.

Guidelines for Talking with Others

- Will telling this person about the affair ruin his or her long-term relationship with my partner?
- Will this person be able to respect my request for confidentiality?
- What specifically do I want from this person?
- If I'm looking for advice, can this person be objective and not just take my side?

Will Telling This Person Ruin His or Her Long-Term Relationship with My Partner?

Particularly if you're the injured partner, you may want to tell your parents, siblings, or friends about what your partner has done and the hurtful effects on you. Sharing such information is one way of eliciting support; it's also a way of expressing your own anger. But before talking with family or friends about your partner's affair, think about how your comments might impact your family member's or friend's relationship with your partner in the future. Although right now you may feel so hurt and angry at your partner that you can't imagine a future together, over time you may feel differently and decide to rebuild your relationship with your partner or continue your marriage. Although *you* might be able to recover from the injury of your partner's affair, will your family member or friend also be able to rebuild a relationship with your partner? We know of numerous families who have been permanently damaged after siblings or parents learned of an in-law's extramarital affair. Despite their best intentions, family members are sometimes unable to move beyond anger or resentment toward a partner who brought such pain to someone they love. We've also seen cases in which the participating partner becomes aware that the injured partner's parents or siblings know what has happened and then feels shame or intense awkwardness that makes it very difficult to interact with the injured partner's family in the future.

Openly discussing an affair with family members and friends not only has the potential to disrupt their relationship with your partner, but may also make it more difficult for you to talk with your family or friends about your relationship in the future. If you and your partner stay together, your family or friends might not support your decision. And if you have other struggles with your partner in the future, it may be difficult to discuss them with your family or friends because they no longer support your marriage.

If you've already talked with a family member or friend about the affair and your partner knows you've done so, it can sometimes be helpful if you and your partner get together with that person and attempt to rebuild the friend's or family member's relationship with your partner. Even if you and your partner decide to separate or divorce, it may be important for your partner to maintain an amicable relationship with your family, particularly if you have children. Although we've seen some extended families work through the painful consequences of an affair together and restore the close relationships they enjoyed previously, we've observed many more cases in which extended family members' knowledge of an affair made it far more difficult for a couple to restore their own relationship. So think carefully about the long-term implications of talking with family or close friends about the affair, recognizing that your own feelings about your partner and your relationship may change in unexpected ways over the coming months.

Will This Person Be Able to Respect My Request for Confidentiality?

You may wish to tell only a few select family members and friends about your affair, anticipating their support or assistance. However, it's important that you also consider whether they will honor your wish for confidentiality. Breaches of confidentiality occur for many reasons. For example, in many families or friendship circles, there's an informal rule that important personal information can and should be shared. Often this information is conveyed in the following way: "Mary told me something very confidential, and she doesn't want anyone else to know. But I thought you needed to know. So don't say anything about it to anyone, okay?" In this way your confidence can end up being shared with a whole host of individuals. If that doesn't seem acceptable to you, think carefully about whom to tell. If people are likely to find out, then you may wish to tell them directly rather than having the information presented second-hand, with all the possibilities of misinformation and distortion. This informal communication pattern among family members or friends is one reason that many people decide to talk about the details of what they're experiencing to professionals instead.

What Specifically Do I Want from This Person?

In choosing which family members or friends to inform, decide first whether you believe they're entitled to know or you'd like some kind of support. If you're looking for support, are you looking for emotional support, for advice, or for other assistance with practical issues or demands? You might turn to different people for different types of support. For example, with friends or family members, you may want primarily emotional support. What you may need is a good shoulder to lean on, someone who understands you and will just listen. This person might be someone to be around when you can "let down" so you don't have to endure this pain by yourself.

There are probably other people whom you're likely to seek out for advice or strategic assistance. For example, you might want the name of a mental health professional or a member of the clergy with whom to talk about your current difficulties, or you may want professional advice from a financial consultant or attorney. (We'll consider the subject of seeking outside professional help further in Chapter 5.) Friends and family members often can be valuable referral sources for you. You might approach a family member or friend for assistance with specific tasks that aren't being accomplished during this time of relationship crisis, such as help with child care, meals, or transportation. You might be in a financial bind and need someone to help. Or you might need someone to help you consider decisions you're facing and decide to talk with a friend or family member whose judgment you particularly value and respect.

Can This Person Be Objective and Not Just Take My Side?

Family members and friends typically see it as their responsibility to support you during a crisis and to see things from your perspective. Consequently, they may tell you how justified you are in feeling as you do and join you in "partner bashing." In fact, research suggests that when maritally distressed women talk to other women who are having marital problems, their conversations about their partners become more negative than when they talk to friends who are happy in their marriages. In other words, your family members or friends can't be totally objective in how they experience your marital situation. Their relationships with you and their own life circumstances will influence how they respond to your situation.

We've seen many examples in which family and friends basically tell an injured partner, "Ditch the jerk and make life as miserable as possible for him (her)." In essence, they're angry about what's happened to you and they want you not to be hurt further by someone who's violated your trust. Although both you and your family and friends might be focusing on negative aspects of your relationship that are so obvious right now, for most people ending a marriage also involves losing much that is good. It's easy to focus on the pain resulting from this affair right now, but you may lose sight of what your relationship has provided in the past and what it might be able to provide at some point again in the future. Only you—not your family member or friend—will have to live with the consequences of whatever long-term decisions you make about your relationship. *So be very careful about placing too much weight on any advice you receive, no matter how well intended.*

Also be aware that if you seek advice from family or friends, they may be upset with you if you don't follow it. Some people seem to believe that if you ask for their advice, you should follow it. They may think that you're too distraught to see the situation clearly and believe that they know what's best for you. Be clear with family and friends that although you may seek out and value their input, there are complicated decisions ahead of you that only you can make. Ask them to respect your final decision, even if it's not consistent with their advice.

Your family and friends can support you in many valuable ways through this difficult time. Research indicates that social support can help to decrease emotional and physical upset during a time of great stress. Although women tend to seek out social support for relationship problems more naturally than men, both men and women can benefit from such support. If you're thoughtful about the friends and family members to whom you turn, if you think about what you want from each of these relationships and carefully consider both the short- and long-term consequences of disclosing the affair, you can benefit from being supported by people who care about you.

What's Next?

Look over the exercises on the following pages, and consider which of these may apply to your own situation. Some of the challenges you're facing in dealing with others depend on the unique circumstances of your own situation, such as whether the affair has ended and whether you have children. Other decisions, such as whom to tell about the affair and for what purposes, are shared by nearly everyone struggling to recover from an affair. Use these exercises to help you translate the principles and ideas we've presented in this chapter into specific decisions and actions.

Then go on to Chapter 5, where we'll help you consider how to care for yourself during this difficult time. You and your partner have a lot of work ahead of you to recover from this affair, whether you do it individually or together. To get through this period, you'll need all the strength and emotional resilience you can muster. Although the emotional support of family and friends can help, the strength you'll need requires you to care for yourself. In Chapter 5, we'll help you consider ways of promoting your own emotional and physical well-being.

——————————— Exercises ———————————

Because everyone's situation is different, not all of these exercises may apply to you—so complete the ones that fit your situation.

• *If you and your partner are working through this book together:* Each of you should think about your own personal opinions on these matters. Then use these exercises to share your thoughts and feelings about these issues and decide what to do.

• *If you're working through the book alone:* If your partner is willing to talk with you about these matters, ask for a time to talk about relating to other people and use the following exercises to structure your conversations. If your partner is unwilling to discuss these issues with you, you'll need to decide on your own what to do, but whenever possible, inform your partner about your plans.

EXERCISE 4.1. HOW DO WE DEAL WITH THE OUTSIDE PERSON?

In setting limits, consider three different issues: (1) the method of communicating with the outside person, (2) the settings for interactions, and (3) what is to be discussed. You might also need to take action to prevent this person from interfering in your lives.

Method of Communication

Do you want to terminate communication with the outside person completely in all ways? Are certain kinds of communication acceptable? If so, what amounts and for what reasons?

Discuss various ways of communicating between the outside person and the individual who had the affair and decide what is acceptable. Is any form of communication acceptable, such as face-to-face, telephone, or e-mail? For what purpose? For example:

> "We've agreed that you're not to have any form of contact with the other person whatsoever. If the outside person sends you an e-mail, you'll ignore it. If that person calls, you'll hang up immediately. If you run into each other, you won't acknowledge or speak."

Or alternatively, you might agree on the following:

> "If the other person contacts you by e-mail, it's okay for you to respond one time, saying never to contact you again. Then you'll ignore all future e-mail messages."

If the affair is ongoing, you still need to discuss what limits are acceptable for now and how these limits will change over time. For example:

> "We've agreed that this outside relationship cannot continue long-term. You'll have two months to decide whether you plan to end that relationship or ours. In the meantime, you're not to take any phone calls here or send e-mail messages from home; it's just too upsetting. You also have agreed to be honest and inform me about your contacts with the outside person. In one week, we'll reassess whether I can live with this arrangement. It will be very hard."

Settings for Communication

Given the circumstances, some interaction with the outside person may be unavoidable. You need to decide how to handle interaction in various settings.

Discuss whether it's acceptable for your partner to interact with the outside person in certain settings and what limits to set. For example:

> "Because you work with this person, I know you can't totally avoid him [her]. We've agreed that it's okay to say hello if you pass the person in the hall or have a group meeting with that person. However, we've also agreed that you won't have any meetings with just the two of you, either in the office or outside—for example, no lunches or coffee breaks one-on-one."

Content of Communication

If you and your partner agree that some forms of communication with the outside person are acceptable, you need to specify what you will and will not discuss with the outside person. Conversations about business are quite different from those about how much you care about each other.

Decide what types of conversation are acceptable, if any. For example:

> "We've agreed that you can discuss business issues, but that's all. You're not to discuss your former relationship with each other or how you feel about each other."

Additional Steps to Set Limits

You may find that the outside person is reluctant or unwilling to stay out of your lives. If so, you might need to take additional action, such as changing your telephone number, consulting with a lawyer, changing jobs, or even moving to another community.

Discuss what additional steps, if any, you need to take to limit this person's involvement in your lives. For example:

> "We will contact our lawyer and ask her to send a letter to the outside person, informing him [her] that he [she] is to have no further con-

tact with any member of our family. If the person doesn't comply, our next step will be to contact the police regarding harassment."

EXERCISE 4.2. WHAT DO WE TELL OUR CHILDREN AND HOW DO WE MINIMIZE THE IMPACT ON THEM?

If you haven't already done so, both you and your partner should read through the section in this chapter on interacting with children and then work through this exercise. Your children's welfare will best be served if you and your partner collaborate on making decisions and implementing them.

What and How to Tell the Children

How much information or detail should you provide your children about the conflict between their parents? What might they already know, or be likely to find out, about the affair or its consequences for your relationship? Will you and your partner talk with your children together or separately? Can you talk with all your children at the same time, or do you need to talk with them individually because of their very different ages? In considering these issues, focus on helping your children understand the consequences of this conflict for them. Tell them what is likely to change and what is likely to remain the same in their own lives.

Decide what you need to convey to your children and how you want to communicate it. For example:

"We've agreed to meet with the children together and to let them know that Mom and Dad are having some difficulties in getting along right now, but that we're getting some help in trying to make things better. We've also agreed not to make any direct or indirect comments about the affair itself."

Minimizing Disruptions to the Family Routine

How can you maintain continuity in your children's lives as much as possible? Will you continue to have meals together? Will both parents continue to be involved in child care, attending school functions, and participating in other family events outside the home? If you're living separately for now, how will you manage visits to extended family or financial matters, such as buying school clothes or paying for college tuition? What other routines in your children's lives could be affected by what's going on in your own relationship right now, and what steps can you take to minimize these disruptions?

Discuss how the current distress in your relationship could affect family routines or other aspects of your children's lives and reach decisions about how to minimize these disruptions. For example:

> "We've agreed to have family meals together and for both of us to participate in our children's school and extracurricular activities. We've agreed during these times not to discuss the affair and to interact as constructively as possible. For now, we've agreed to wait one month before reaching a decision about how to deal with summer vacation."

EXERCISE 4.3. WHOM ELSE DO WE TELL?

Who needs to know about your current relationship problem in order to deal with certain consequences of it? You child's teacher or your financial adviser? A family member with whom you were going to spend a holiday? Does anyone need to know specifically about the affair, such as your physician so that you can be tested for sexually transmitted diseases? Whom do you want to tell about your relationship problems so that you can receive practical support—for example, perhaps a next-door neighbor who could help with transportation for you or the children? Whom do you want to approach for emotional support? Perhaps a family member or close friend? What limits do you want to place on how much you disclose? Could disclosing the affair place you, your partner, or this individual in a difficult position in the long term?

Be clear about what you want from the individual, whether this person is appropriate for this need, whether confiding in this person could hamper your recovery as a couple in the long term, and whether the person is likely to respect your wishes for confidentiality. Be sure to set your own limits on whom to talk with and how much information to share.

Decide whom you want to talk with and how much you want to disclose. For example:

"I want to talk with my best friend, Mary, about the affair because I value her judgment and her emotional support. If other friends ask me about what's going on, I want to disclose only that my partner and I are having some relationship problems but are working on them. For now, I would prefer that neither my family nor my partner's family know about our relationship problems. I'm willing to reevaluate this decision a month from now."

5

>>> ————————————————————————

How Do We Care
for Ourselves?

Brian's life turned upside down after he discovered Katherine's affair. He couldn't sleep, he couldn't eat, and his normal routines were completely disrupted. His emotions swung wildly from numbness to intense anxiety and depression. Normally he turned to Katherine for help, but now she seemed like a stranger. He had no idea how to get his emotions and life back under control.

Katherine was consumed with guilt over her affair, lying awake at night, tormented by thoughts of the pain she had caused her family. At the same time, she was furious at Brian for the pain he had caused her by abandoning her for his countless golf tournaments. When they tried to discuss her affair, this combination of pain and anger was so unbearable that Katherine would often lose control and scream at Brian. These outbursts only made things worse, but neither of them knew how to break out of the cycle.

When you're worried about an affair and whether you can survive, thinking about eating well and getting exercise can seem trivial. Yet that's what we're asking you to do in this chapter. The days and weeks following the discovery of an affair can be chaotic and emotionally traumatic. You can barely get through the day and manage the work you have to do. You need all the strength you can get. At the same time, taking care of yourself is all the more difficult in times of acute stress.

Because we understand how critical self-care is but also know that right now it may seem like just one more heavy burden, we ask you to read this chapter with three goals in mind, with no pressure to achieve them. Just think about them.

1. Come to see self-care as critical to your recovery, even if you don't feel you can take the time to pursue it or don't feel you deserve to take the time for yourself because of your guilt, shame, or lowered self-esteem.
2. Figure out how to make it through the day in a healthy manner. Identify ways you can increase your current levels of self-care in specific domains—physical, social, emotional, and spiritual—all of which will help you manage stress better.
3. Consider whether you need to bring in additional sources of help. We'll tell you where you can find them.

Why Is Self-Care Important?

First, adequate self-care is essential to combat the effects of stress. The discovery or disclosure of an affair typically creates high, sustained stress for both partners. Paradoxically, just when we most need additional emotional, physical, and social resources, we're often least likely to engage in behaviors designed to renew these resources. For example, just when you feel exhausted and most in need of a good night's sleep, you may find yourself lying awake at night, worrying about the future or reviewing every detail of the past to try to understand what went wrong. Lack of sleep means more exhaustion and less resilience. Plenty of scientific research has demonstrated that anxiety and depression wreak havoc on people's ability to sleep, creating a double whammy because the less sleep you get, the more prone to anxiety and depression you become. Depression and anxiety may also disrupt your appetite, leading you to pick at your food or even feel repulsed by the thought of eating. Or the same emotions may drive you to overeat or indulge in "comfort foods" that tend to be high in fat and calories and low in nutritional value. The disruption of normal routines and increased stress may also lead you to put off your normal exercise routine, depriving you of the emotional and physical benefits of regular physical activity.

The affair may also disrupt important aspects of your social and spiritual life. For example, your worry about others discovering the problems you and your partner are having may lead you to avoid friends and family. If most of your friends are other couples that you and your partner have enjoyed together, you may now find yourself isolated. Or if you and your partner or the outside affair person have attended the same church or synagogue, you may avoid going there now. You may feel even more isolated if you and your partner have specifically agreed that you don't want anyone else to know about the affair. Countless studies have shown that social support has a major impact on emotional, psychological, and even physical health. Consequently, increased social isolation may only heighten the anxiety, depression, or other emotional turmoil that follows the discovery of an affair.

You can end up feeling particularly isolated if your partner has always been a major source of emotional support for you. Perhaps you used to discuss events of the day together and you valued your partner's opinions. Or perhaps you didn't talk often, but you believed that your partner would always be there for you. Now, when you most need emotional support and caring, you may feel unable to turn to your partner. If you can't turn to your partner, and you're reluctant to turn to others because of agreements to keep the affair confidential, where can you find the support you need to get through the day? We'll tell you where later in the chapter. For now the point is that you may find yourself needing to take care of yourself in ways you haven't needed to do so before.

Second, failure to take care of yourself will inevitably make things worse. Research on the mind–body connection clearly shows that failure to eat well and get adequate sleep leads to a decreased ability to regulate one's emotions. How often have you noticed that you or other members of your family become more irritable during the hour before dinner? Or how many times have you snapped at a friend or coworker, only to apologize later and blame it on lack of sleep? Again, research confirms that lack of sleep impairs awareness, clouds decision-making ability, and leads to more difficulty in coping with strong feelings. Lack of sleep, poor nutrition, inadequate social support—all lead to increased emotional and physical difficulties. So the bottom line is this: *If you don't take care of yourself during this difficult recovery process, you're likely to find both you and your relationship getting worse.* Good self-care helps to build up your resilience and strengthen you for the hard work that lies ahead in rebuilding your life after the affair.

How Do I Get Through the Day?

Attending to Physical Needs

You may have recognized yourself in some of our earlier descriptions—sleeping too little, eating too little or too much, or failing to get adequate exercise. Even if you believe you're managing these functions well, take time to read through the physical self-care strategies discussed below. That you need sleep, nutritious food, and other contributors to good physical health will come as no news to you, but you may find that there are ways you can attend to your physical needs better, now or in the future. Exercise 5.1 will help you do this.

Sleep and Rest

The emotional turmoil that accompanies the discovery or disclosure of an affair interferes with your ability to rest. Simply being anxious or depressed can disrupt sleep. To make matters worse, the strategies that many of us try to compensate for lost sleep actually make things worse. Staying up late so you won't lie awake staring at the ceiling, staying up all night because there's no point in trying to sleep when you can't, taking naps during the day, and single-handedly supporting your local coffee shop may seem helpful in the short run, but these strategies are also likely to maintain your sleep difficulties in the long run. Instead, work to learn and follow good sleep practices.

How? First, avoid taking naps or limit them to 20 minutes in the morning or early afternoon. Also avoid caffeine, alcohol, or other mood-altering substances—all of which are likely to interfere with your sleep patterns. Try to get up and go to bed at the same times every day and develop a relaxing "winding-down" routine before bed. This routine could include a warm bath, a relaxing book (probably not this book!), soft music, or gentle stretching exercises. The goal is to get yourself into a relaxed frame of mind before bed. If you can't fall asleep after 20 minutes, instead of lying in bed worrying, get up and spend 20 minutes doing some quiet activity such as playing solitaire or reading a nonstimulating book. Avoid watching TV, because it's easy to get caught up in late-night talk shows or movie reruns instead of falling asleep. After 20 minutes, go back to bed and try again. You may need to repeat this pattern several times.

Following these strategies should eventually help you break the anxious no-sleep cycle. If not, it's important to avoid over-the-counter sleeping pills; they're likely to cause a rebound effect and continue your sleeping problems once you discontinue their use. If you're still unable to restore a nearly normal sleeping pattern for yourself after applying these strategies, consider discussing your sleep problems with your physician and trying a prescription sleep medication on a trial basis. Once sleep is restored with medication, the strategies described above often maintain good sleep patterns without medication even in times of increased stress.

Nutrition

Healthy eating is literally one way to nurture yourself during this difficult time. Skipping meals or bingeing on junk food once in a great while may not be harmful; the problem occurs when it becomes a habit or continual response. If your blood sugar and protein levels drop too low, your ability to regulate your emotions also decreases, causing you to act impulsively and probably more intensely than you would if you were well rested and well fed. Even if you're not aware that you're hungry but you've gone several hours without adequate nutrition, you're probably at greater risk for being irritable or jumpy. In fact, if you're depressed, relying on your appetite as a cue for when to eat can cause problems because severe depression may limit your appetite and mild to moderate depression may increase it. Instead, learning what your body needs to perform adequately and then planning when and what to eat throughout the day is probably a more effective strategy. Taking time at regular intervals to eat some fruit, consume some protein, and provide your body with some form of complex carbohydrate should help you keep your emotions on a more even keel. If you're uncertain about how to pursue a balanced diet, there are plenty of good books on this topic at your bookstore or public library.

Exercise

When people's lives feel chaotic or stressful, their regular exercise routines are often the first thing sacrificed when, instead, exercise should probably be one of the top priorities. You may feel too tired or too worn out by daily stressors or by the intense emotions you're feeling to even contemplate exercising. The lure of the couch may be tough to resist. Alternatively, although you might want to exercise, you may not believe you deserve or can afford to take the time away from your family or your other responsibilities to pursue it. *Our view is: You can't afford not to.* Exercise has been shown to be an effective mood regulator; several studies have shown that people are able to significantly reduce their feelings of anxiety and depression through regular, moderate exercise. Exercise has also been shown to increase endorphins, the hormones released when we engage in pleasurable activities such as eating chocolate or engaging in sexual activity. So you owe it to yourself to engage in regular exercise, even if you do so only to renew your resources so that you can give more to others around you the next day.

If exercise hasn't been part of your routine before, start with small goals—for example, taking a brisk 30-minute walk three times a week. Schedule times for exercise when you're least likely to be distracted or interrupted, just as you would for other vital tasks. Some people play their favorite music or watch the news on TV while exercising; others work out with a friend who can provide encouragement and accountability. Variety in exercise routines (for example, exercising different muscle groups on different days—or walking in different neighborhoods or even in different directions around the block!) can help to prevent boredom. Set modest goals, record your progress, and don't let a lapse of a day or two prevent you from starting up your routine again. Start today—at least for 15 minutes—and then go from there.

Health

Physical illness and related health problems also reduce your emotional resilience and decrease your ability to cope with individual and relationship challenges. If you've recently developed physical problems or have been putting off getting medical attention for an ongoing condition, don't delay any longer in seeing your physician; make an appointment today. Along the same lines, take any medications you're supposed to be taking as prescribed. Taking time to visit your physician and complying with treatment will help you deal more effectively with your emotional difficulties in the long run. Like many of us, you may tend to ignore physical concerns until there's a crisis. Consider this a crisis of a different kind that demands extra care of your health!

Similarly, making healthy choices to limit alcohol, caffeine, and other nonprescription psychoactive substances is also important. Alcohol, caffeine, and nicotine can significantly interfere with your ability to get a good night's sleep and can make your existing mood problems worse. Caffeine and nicotine are likely to make you feel more physically aroused, which can lead to greater emotional irritability and difficulty in regulating your negative emotions. For example, you may become more likely to snap at your partner, particularly if you're already stressed. In addition, alcohol is a depressant and will make any depressive tendencies worse; because of its tendency to suppress inhibitions, alcohol may also make you more likely to say and do things you'll later regret. Although all of these substances may appear to offer short-term relief from painful feelings, in the long term their use may backfire and increase the likelihood of your continuing to feel emotionally drained or out of control.

Attending to Social Needs

Scientists studying stress have found without a doubt that social support not only can help decrease emotional turmoil but also actually promotes physical health during times of stress. Now more than ever, when you may very well feel isolated, at least from your partner, close friends and family members can provide you with care and concern, serve as sounding boards, help you talk through your feelings, provide an emotional buffer against deep loneliness, possibly offer reassurance or hope, and encourage you to take care of yourself by joining you in exercise, healthy meals, or other activities that help to offset at least some of the pain you're experiencing.

The important thing to remember about seeking such support is to know what you want from which people. Maybe there are only one or two individuals you would want to talk with about the affair, but others whom you might tell that you and your partner have stopped going out together with other couples for the time being so they'll be more inclined to invite you to spend time together one-on-one. Do you have a larger circle of people who aren't confidants but whom you might enjoy spending time with to get temporary relief from thinking about the affair? You might find social support in spending more time in group functions at your church, your children's school, or your neighborhood.

Denise wanted to hide under her bedcovers when she first discovered Eric's affair. She was sure his betrayal was written all over her face. She withdrew from her regular book group and stopped attending church but soon noticed that her isolation was deepening her feelings of despair. So she arranged a few lunches with close friends who were sensitive and supportive. Two of her friends invited her to a girls' night out at an art gallery, which Denise found herself enjoying immensely. The next day, her future didn't seem as bleak as it had the day before, and she vowed to make these outings regular events.

Attending to Emotional Needs

Anxiety, depression, and anger take a toll on your physical health, get in the way of meeting your day-to-day responsibilities, and often intrude on your interactions with your partner in ways that make recovery more difficult. You can ignore these feelings or try to bury them, but rarely without health consequences or fallout that will affect relationships in the future. Instead, consider the following strategies for making times of emotional upset more manageable, and use Exercise 5.2 to tailor these strategies to your own needs.

Taking a Long-Term Perspective

Chang often talked at length about how painful Ming's affair had been for him. These conversations made Ming feel guilty, and she often responded with angry outbursts, accusing Chang of driving her to have the affair. Although Ming's outbursts were sometimes successful in ending Chang's prolonged discussions about her affair, the long-term consequences of Ming's reactions were clearly destructive. Chang withdrew into angry silence. Ming's accusations about his causing her affair led him to feel defensive and less willing to examine his own role in their relationship. They became mired in a destructive cycle of attacks and counterattacks that interfered with their recovery from the affair.

When your feelings in the moment seem overwhelming but your reactions to those feelings seem to make things worse, carefully consider your long-term goals for yourself and your relationship. Try to keep these goals in mind when you interact with your partner and then work at responding in ways that are consistent with those goals. If your long-term goal is to rebuild your relationship, be aware that losing your temper and repeatedly lashing out at your partner won't help. If your long-term goal is to help your partner feel emotionally more secure, recognize that walking away each time your partner expresses upset feelings is counterproductive.

Tolerating distress and refraining from destructive reactions in the moment, although difficult, often become easier when you consciously remind yourself of your long-term individual and relationship goals.

Using Self-Talk

By "self-talk" we mean talking to yourself so you can stay on track and focused on what's helpful to you and your relationship. Reminding yourself of long-term goals is a type of self-talk that can help you manage your emotions. Self-talk can also help you get through strong feelings in the moment: "Okay, this feels really bad right now. But that doesn't mean it's always going to feel this way. If I can try to get through this one day at a time, eventually things can get better." And it can help you assert personal control over your own behavior: "I'm not going to let that argument ruin the weekend. I can't let it take over my whole life. There are still good things in my life, and I need to enjoy them."

Self-talk can also help you challenge false beliefs and other thoughts that may not be serving you well. Research clearly shows that once a relationship starts to go sour, people often interpret a partner's behavior in the most negative possible way. Let's say you get home late and your partner asks, "Where were you?" You could assume your partner is expressing suspicion—or you could use self-talk to step back and consider whether this was actually an expression of interest or concern for your safety. Once your partner has had an affair, you might be likely to interpret much of your partner's behavior as selfish or deceitful. That's a trap you need to avoid; seeing your partner as entirely bad or without any good qualities just makes things worse. Challenge your interpretations by asking yourself, "Why am I upset? Are there other explanations for what my partner just did or said that would be less upsetting?" You may subsequently decide that your initial interpretation was correct, but you can't even *consider* less hurtful explanations if you don't challenge yourself in this way.

Self-talk can be put to lots of constructive use, but you should also be aware that all of us engage in internal dialogues that may be *creating or increasing* negative emotions. If you're anxious, you may be telling yourself that this situation is intolerable and will never get better. If you're angry, you may be focusing on how terrible your partner is. If you're depressed, you may be blaming yourself for the affair or feeling hopeless about the future. It's important to step back from your feelings and examine any self-talk that may be contributing to them. Is there a difference between your partner's doing something profoundly hurtful and being a horrible person? Did your own contributions to relationship problems in the past really make you responsible for your partner's affair? Are you likely to feel this miserable for the rest of your life? Consider other people you know who've had serious relationship problems or have ended a marriage. Are all of their lives ruined, with no pleasure at all anymore?

Using constructive self-talk, you may decide that although you've played some role in your relationship problems, you're not responsible for your partner's decision to have an affair. Or you may recognize that although your life feels shattered and it's difficult to *feel* hopeful, in reality many partners find a way to work through crises together or go on to build satisfying lives separately. When you step back and challenge some of your negative thoughts, chances are you'll come up with a more balanced view of the situation that brings your emotions to a more bearable level.

"Riding Out" Your Feelings

Intensely painful feelings often feel like they'll never end. But when scientists have taken a closer look, they've found they are often self-limited and come in waves. As strong as these emotions may feel in the present moment, if you "ride out the wave," the feelings will often reach a peak and then diminish on their own. People sometimes prolong their distress by berating themselves for having their feelings, reminding themselves of how unfair it is that they should have to feel this way, or demanding that the partner do something to make the feelings better. If instead you can imagine these intense feelings as a wave and anticipate that they will eventually decline, you may feel better equipped to get through the most difficult part of your immediate experience. The increased emotional distance can also allow you to think more clearly about what your feelings are and what triggered them.

> Rachael had considerable trouble managing both her anger and her anxiety when she and her husband, Dan, argued. Feeling acutely distressed, she would sometimes pursue the argument and escalate their conflict until one of them pushed or shoved the other. Once Rachael learned that emotions were like waves and that she could ride them out until they decreased to a more tolerable level on their own, she was able to stop her demands that Dan do something to

make her feel better, which in turn had been provoking even stronger arguments.

Learning to ride out difficult feelings can also be helpful for participating partners who sometimes struggle with waves of missing the outside person. If you've ended an affair and are committed to rebuilding your marriage, but sometimes still have strong feelings for the outside person and urges to renew contact, redirecting your thoughts or activities elsewhere to ride out these feelings can be an effective way of dealing with your own emotional needs. We've worked with participating partners who have misinterpreted such feelings as an indication that a relationship with the outside person was "meant to be," only to regret responding to these feelings later on.

Venting

Recognizing that feelings sometimes come in waves isn't always enough to make them tolerable. At times you may be able to ride out intense emotions, but at other times you may need strategies for "skimming" or "taking the edge off" your feelings to bring them down to a more manageable level. "Venting" is one way of making feelings more manageable. Letter writing (see Chapter 3) is one way to vent your feelings. Letters written for the sake of venting are destroyed after being written so that they provide an outlet for your strongest feelings without causing worry about their impact on your partner or anyone else.

Another means of venting is to talk with someone you trust to hear your uncensored feelings without reacting to them and without interpreting them as necessarily reflecting how you *usually* feel. A very good friend can serve as an outlet for venting, by phone or in person, as long as you choose the right person (see Chapter 4 and the section "Attending to Social Needs" in this chapter). And don't overdo it; even good friends can grow tired of long or frequent venting sessions.

Gaining Distance

Some of the techniques we've described involve gaining distance from your feelings. Adopting a long-term perspective helps you get some emotional distance from what's happening in the immediate moment. Self-talk helps you take a step back from negative thoughts or feelings and see the bigger picture. You can also gain some distance by using the time-out techniques discussed in Chapter 3 or by distracting yourself from thinking about the affair. Going for a walk, reading the newspaper or watching TV, or engaging in a hobby may provide just enough relief in the short run to allow you to manage your feelings and then address them more effectively either individually or with your partner. We're not proposing that you avoid addressing problems, but there are times when you and your partner need to get away from them. Distracting yourself with fun or engaging activities can be a healthy way to cope when problems feel overwhelming.

Increasing Positive Experiences

Good emotional self-care involves more than managing negative feelings; it also involves increasing positive experiences. When people are anxious and depressed, they're more likely to withdraw and stop pursuing pleasurable, fun, or rewarding activities. Your emotional distress may exhaust you to the point that all you feel like doing is lying on the couch. However, if that's all you do, you're likely to end up feeling worse. Inactivity tends to increase depression and isolation, which makes you feel even less like doing anything pleasurable. This downward spiral is difficult to escape if you continue to do things only when you "feel like it." Instead, it's important that you commit to doing something good for yourself on a regular basis, even if it's just a relaxing bath at the end of the day, a weekly massage, or meeting one of your friends for a game of basketball after work. Just as with regular exercise, committing to pleasurable activities is critical to ensuring that you'll have the emotional reserves you need to get through this tough time and to treat the people around you well. In other words, you owe it to *them* to do this for yourself.

Attending to Spiritual Needs

During times of crisis many people draw on their spiritual life, and others find it helpful to deepen their spirituality if this part of their life has been lacking. Attending to your spiritual needs may promote a feeling of inner strength or help in examining the affair from a broader perspective. An affair raises profoundly difficult questions for both partners. What do I value the most in life? How do I reconcile what I value with how I actually behave? How do I find the strength to get through this excruciating experience? How can I manage this profound guilt or rage? How do I find meaning or purpose in this crisis? What do I believe about forgiveness or reconciliation? Exploring your personal spiritual life may help you in examining these critical questions.

Spiritual self-care often involves:

- Renewing or increasing your involvement in a church or synagogue.
- Pursuing prayer, meditation, or other means of inspiration.
- Expressing your spiritual life through art, poetry, or service to others.
- Developing a relationship with a spiritual mentor or adviser.

In addition to finding direction in considering difficult issues or decisions, many people gain strength and comfort from their spiritual life. Various studies have shown that people reporting an active spiritual life have lower rates of depression, anxiety, and stress-related health problems. Although the reasons for these effects aren't fully understood, explanations have emphasized individuals' sense of belonging to a larger community, confidence in a benevolent higher power, and ability to view current crises in a broader context and life meaning.

An individual's spirituality is a profoundly personal experience. In fact, you may decide that spirituality is unrelated to how you care for yourself. However, if spirituality has been an important part of your life in the past, or if you believe that it might be helpful to you during this particularly difficult time, we strongly encourage you to draw on your spiritual life in whatever ways may serve you best. Some people may renew their involvement in a local church, synagogue, or other religious group. For other persons, pursuing their spirituality involves meditation or prayer. You might find strength, courage, or direction in reading inspirational accounts of other persons' survival of traumatic experiences or triumphs over immense challenges to achieve a difficult goal. Some people express their spiritual life through art, poetry, or service to others. And still others develop a mentoring or supportive relationship with a spiritual adviser. We don't presume to tell you *how* to attend to your spiritual needs. But we do encourage you to consider your spiritual life as one important way of caring for yourself.

Should I Seek Professional Help Just for Me?

Deborah fell apart after discovering Victor's affair. Her initial shock and anger gradually turned into endless numbness. Weeks went by, but she simply couldn't get herself to function. She stayed in bed for hours at a time, staring at the wall. Her job began to suffer, and eventually her supervisor told her that unless she returned to work and managed her responsibilities better, she would be fired. Deborah needed to pull herself together, but she had no idea how.

When Should I Seek Professional Help?

Although there's no simple answer to this question, a general guideline to follow is to **pursue separate help for yourself if:**

- Your responses to the affair are so acutely intense in the short term that they could result in serious harm to yourself or others.
- Your emotional distress continues over an extended period of time at a level that prevents individual or relationship recovery.

Signs that you might benefit from outside assistance include the following:

- *Severe or persistent depression.* Thoughts about suicide or actual attempts to harm yourself. Severe disruption of your sleep, eating, or other physical self-care that could lead to negative consequences for your health. Profound and unshakable feelings of hopelessness, worthlessness, or guilt. Repeated crying spells that last 30 minutes or longer. Nearly complete loss of interest in daily activities involving work, home, friends, or family on an ongoing basis.
- *Severe or persistent anxiety.* Overwhelming fear or worry that brings emotional or physical exhaustion. Inability to concentrate or think clearly. Acute physiological arousal resulting in severe headaches, muscle tension, stomach upset, or chest pains. Recurrent episodes of panic or chronic dread that continue despite efforts to engage in emotional self-care.
- *Rage or physical aggression against others.* Uncontrolled verbal or physical aggression directed toward your partner, the outside affair person,

or others. Acts of retaliation against your partner that you later regret, such as destruction of property. Sudden outbursts of anger toward persons uninvolved in the affair, such as your children or coworkers.

• *Behaviors harmful to yourself.* Actions that provide pleasure or relief in the short run but may harm you in the long run. For example, excessive use of alcohol or other substances to influence your mood, spending sprees that create financial hardship, or having an affair of your own as a way of "getting even."

• *Inability to reach critical decisions.* Inability to reach decisions for yourself about how to manage this crisis in the short term—such as how to confront your partner or the outside affair person, what to tell the children, or whether to continue living together. Or inability to approach longer-term decisions—for example, how long to tolerate your partner's affair if it hasn't ended, or whether to commit to restoring this relationship or move on separately.

If one or more of these descriptions apply to you, it's important to get separate help for yourself. You might also decide to seek outside assistance even if your difficulties don't appear as severe as those described above. Getting outside help isn't self-indulgent, and it doesn't reflect moral or character weakness; it's about survival and about becoming healthy again for the sake of those persons you care about and who care about you. Among the benefits that outside professionals may provide are greater experience or expertise in dealing with relationship problems, ability to offer specific resources such as medication, greater capacity to remain objective, and commitment to confidentiality. Exercise 5.3 can help you decide whether to seek professional help.

How Can I Find Help, and What Should I Expect?

In surveys about whom people turn to in times of emotional distress, the most frequently identified professionals are clergy. If you're currently involved in a church or other religious organization, consider requesting counseling from your minister, rabbi, or spiritual adviser. Sometimes religious counselors can be particularly helpful in reaching decisions that incorporate broader spiritual values. They may also offer special support by promoting your prayer life or by suggesting books that integrate spiritual with individual or relationship needs. If you're not currently involved in a church or synagogue or are uncomfortable approaching your own minister or rabbi, but see this kind of assistance as potentially helpful to you, consider asking a trusted friend to recommend a minister, rabbi, or other spiritual leader.

Although churches, synagogues, and individual clergy vary considerably, most have strong values supporting marriage and family life. Knowing this, you may decide that separate help through a church or synagogue doesn't best serve your needs. If you're struggling to reach a decision about whether to leave your partner who's had an affair or whether to continue your affair and leave your marriage, and if you're concerned about whether your minister or rabbi can be entirely objective, you may prefer to seek a nonclergy counselor instead.

Other people may prefer to seek help from a professional in the mental health field. Mental health professionals who provide counseling have diverse backgrounds, levels of training, and areas of expertise. Licensed clinical or counseling psychologists typically have a doctoral degree (PhD or PsyD) and at least five years of training beyond their college or bachelor's degree in working with people who are experiencing emotional and behavioral problems. Social workers are usually licensed with a master's degree (MSW) and have two to three years of training beyond college. Some states also license marital and family therapists with a master's degree (MA or MS) and may certify or license a separate group of professional counselors at the master's degree level. Psychiatrists first receive their training in medicine as physicians (MD) and then pursue a two- to three-year specialized residency in psychiatry; although some psychiatrists provide individual or couple counseling, many emphasize medication as a primary intervention for emotional difficulties.

In addition to these differences in background, professional counselors differ widely in their approaches to individual and relationship problems. Some have extensive training and experience in treating individuals, but little or none in working with couples or families. Some may focus primarily on your communication and current ways of behaving; others might examine relationship patterns in your family or culture; still others may explore underlying needs or conflicts outside your immediate awareness that contribute to current difficulties.

With all these options, how can you make an informed decision about where to get help? One approach is to seek recommendations from individuals in related professions. Your clergyperson or your family physician may know of professional counselors with special expertise in helping people deal with relationship problems. If you live in a community with a college or university, there may be a university-affiliated clinic that offers individual or couple counseling. Or you may be able to obtain information about professionals in the community from the university's department of psychology, college of education, or office of student support services. You may also know of a friend or family member who pursued professional counseling and can suggest someone to see or to call for a recommendation. If all else fails, look through the Yellow Pages of your phone book for listings of the professionals mentioned above, call several of these professionals, ask each to identify the top three or four therapists in the community for dealing with relationship problems, and see if any counselor's name surfaces more than once. Then call that individual, request a five-minute phone conversation to describe your situation, and ask whom that person would recommend.

What's Next?

Complete the exercises on the following pages, which may also give you a better understanding of how to encourage your partner to care for him- or herself. After completing these exercises, you're ready to move on to Chapter 6 and the next stage of recovery. Chapters 6 through 11 are designed to help you explore how this affair came about.

———————————————— **Exercises** ————————————————

EXERCISE 5.1. ATTENDING TO YOUR PHYSICAL NEEDS

Taking care of your basic physical needs means making sure you get adequate sleep, maintain good nutrition, engage in regular exercise, and take care of any physical health problems you're experiencing. Carefully evaluate how you're handling each of these areas. Are you staying up too late or having difficulty falling asleep? Are you skipping meals or eating too much junk food? Have you abandoned regular exercise? Have your current stresses caused health problems or made previous problems worse?

Decide what steps you can take right now to improve your overall physical well-being. For example:

"I'm going to get ready for bed by 10:00 P.M. and read for 30 minutes to relax and help me fall asleep."

Or

"I'm going to take a brisk walk with the dog for 30 minutes each night after dinner."

Or

"I'm going to check with my doctor about the tightness in my chest and occasional difficulties in breathing I've been experiencing."

Write down at least two steps toward better physical self-care you in-tend to implement starting today. In one week, take an honest look at how well you've done. If you've fallen short of your goal, consider what you've let get in the way, and what you could do differently to get on track.

EXERCISE 5.2. MANAGING YOUR EMOTIONS

Strong feelings of anxiety, depression, or anger can become disabling if they're not managed adequately. There are a number of strategies you can pursue on your own to help you to tolerate and manage difficult feel-ings more effectively. Review the guidelines in this chapter for attending to your emotional needs. Which of these strategies might work best for you? For example, how can you use self-talk to calm yourself in times of despair? What methods of venting can you use to reduce the intensity of your emotions and make them more manageable? Beyond managing your negative feelings, how can you increase your positive experiences to provide yourself with greater emotional resilience? How can you draw on spiritual resources to find strength, meaning, or guidance in this crisis?

Decide on strategies for managing your intense negative feelings. For example:

"When I'm starting to feel out of control, I'm going to find a separate space for 20 minutes to challenge my worst fears and remind myself that I can survive this."

Or

"When I feel as though I'm about to explode from thinking about the affair, I'm going to pursue a separate activity to distract myself and get some relief. If that doesn't work, I'll write myself a letter as a way to 'unload' and will then tear it up."

Outline specific steps for increasing your positive experiences. For example:

"I'm going to take 30 minutes each evening to do something for myself—whether it's reading a novel, meditating, fixing a healthy snack, or refinishing the bookcase."

Or

"I'm going to join my church bowling team and enjoy this fellowship with people I like."

As in the previous exercise, write down at least two *steps toward better emotional self-care you intend to implement starting today. Be sure to include at least one strategy for managing negative feelings and one for increasing positive experiences. In one week, take an honest look at how well you've done. If either strategy hasn't worked as well as you had hoped, what could you do to implement that strategy more effectively? What additional or alternative strategies might you use?*

EXERCISE 5.3. DECIDING WHETHER TO SEEK PROFESSIONAL HELP

Consider the potential benefits of getting outside help, either for you individually or for both of you together. You may prefer not to share information about the affair with friends or family members because you lack confidence in their ability to be objective, preserve confidentiality, or respect your decisions down the road if you don't follow their advice. Or your own personal distress or conflicts with your partner may be so intense or complex that you'd prefer the counsel of someone more experienced or specifically trained in dealing with such matters, such as a member of the clergy or a mental health professional. Consider whether you'd prefer to receive counseling for yourself alone, for each of you separately, or for you and your partner together. In some communities, mental health services are offered on a sliding-fee schedule through a public clinic or university-based counseling center; such services might also be provided as a benefit through your insurance or HMO.

Decide what outside professional assistance you might need and explore ways of obtaining it. For example:

> "I'd prefer that my partner and I get some counseling together to help us manage our conflict better and reach some important decisions as a couple. I'll call our minister to see whether he can provide this and, if not, whom he would recommend. If my partner won't join me in these efforts, I'll pursue individual counseling for myself."

Part II

HOW DID THIS HAPPEN?

>>> ──────────────────────────────────────

6

Why Stir Everything Up?

"It's time to put it behind us," Brent said firmly. "We're moving on. I know I did wrong, and I know I won't do it again. Now we need to focus on us and how we're going to be with each other." Anne wanted nothing more than to move on. She wanted to trust Brent with all her heart, and she knew they had both worked hard to get through the initial trauma of his affair. But to Brent, moving on meant no longer discussing the affair. Every time they talked about it, Anne dissolved in tears or exploded in anger, or both, so he believed these discussions simply fed Anne's pain.

Anne, however, kept thinking about the affair, no matter how hard she tried not to. How could he have done this? Had something been missing in their marriage? If so, could she count on him to be faithful the next time they went through a difficult time? Had he been naively seduced by this other woman, who convinced Brent that Anne didn't adequately appreciate him? How could Anne compete with someone who placed no demands on Brent, and why should she try?

Until she was certain that both of them understood how and why his affair had occurred, Anne couldn't feel secure that it wouldn't eventually happen again. She couldn't move on.

If you and your partner have worked successfully through Part I of this book, or even if you've worked through it largely on your own, some of the initial turmoil following the discovery of an affair may now be under better control. Restoring some of the daily routines in your own life and in your relationship, decreasing angry exchanges or reducing some of the emotional distance between you, and taking care of yourselves can bring considerable relief to both of you.

So why stir everything up? Why ask why? Why did this affair happen? How could you or your partner have done this? What went wrong? *The reasons for asking "why" are simple, even if their ramifications are complex:*

- If you're the injured partner, you need to learn as much as you can about why this affair happened to restore the emotional security essential to trust and intimacy.
- If you're the partner who had the affair, you need to explore why this affair happened **because it's what your partner needs**.

We underscored the last phrase above so that both of you will understand that for right now the injured partner's concerns need to take priority. As we said throughout Part I, exploring how the affair came about is necessary to moving on in a healthy way. But a necessary first step is to restore the injured partner's sense of emotional security. The affair shattered that security and threw the injured party completely off balance. Figuring out why it happened is the only way to get the injured party back on solid enough ground to even consider whether a relationship of trust and intimacy can be rebuilt. If you're the participating partner, there are direct benefits for you as well, such as understanding yourself better and making sure you're less likely to be tempted by infidelity again. This exploration involves stirring things up and tolerating more discomfort in the short run. There may be issues in your relationship or aspects of each of you that are difficult to acknowledge and perhaps painful to discuss. We'll help you assess whether you're ready for this work later in the chapter, before you tackle it. But for now, we'll say it one more time: Our 50 years of collective experience with couples struggling after an affair have shown that **coming to a fuller understanding of why an affair occurred is simultaneously the most difficult and also the most important stage of recovery.**

We sometimes describe this stage of recovery as "finding meaning" in the affair. *Finding meaning* involves trying to make sense of something that seems senseless—developing an understanding of something that seems incomprehensible. In searching for meaning, it's important to distinguish between *reasons* and *excuses*—and between *understanding* and *agreement*. If you're the injured person, no number of reasons will excuse your partner's affair. If you're the participating partner in the affair, you may not be asking to be excused. (Most of the participating partners we work with don't expect to be *excused* for their affairs and the hurt they've brought to their partners.) We want you to *understand* why the affair has occurred but not agree with your partner's decision to have an affair. Understanding requires looking at the big picture—or what we call the *context*—for the affair. It involves examining all the factors that contributed to an increased risk, or *vulnerability*, that this affair would occur. None of these factors—individually or collectively—*caused* this affair. Ultimately, *responsibility* for having an affair rests with the person who chooses to engage in the affair, consciously or not, in response to whatever created the risk or vulnerability.

To grasp the difference between assigning responsibility and understanding the context in which the affair happened, think of your relationship as a house that's been burglarized. After a break-in, it's important to examine what made your home vulnerable. Is it in a high-risk neighborhood? Did you take appropriate precautions and keep your home secure? Did you notice strangers lurking about the neighborhood but ignore them? Did you leave valuables out in the open, unwatched, and ready for the taking by some thief waiting for an opportunity? If your home has been burglarized, you're not responsible for the thief's criminal behavior. But if you're going to remain in the home—and even if you move to a new home—you'll feel more secure if you figure out what made your home vulnerable and take deliberate actions to eliminate these risk factors.

Just like the safety of that house, the security of your relationship has been breached. Something precious—your trust and emotional safety—has been violated. A variety of factors could have made your relationship vulnerable. Maybe important parts of your relationship weren't nurtured or protected from outside distractions. Perhaps one of you interacted with outsiders who didn't value your commitment or sexual fidelity to each other. Maybe you missed important warning signs. Frequent arguments may have put distance between you. Whatever the contributing factors were, they didn't *cause* the affair, but they increased your relationship's vulnerability to it. Once you identify these factors, you're in a much better position to decide whether and how to change things. Then you can move forward. Not all couples are ready or willing to accept this challenge.

Both Brent and Anne desperately wanted their marriage to work. But they had different visions of what it would take. When Brent insisted that it was time to stop talking about it, they dropped out of couple therapy, but two months later they were back. Their marriage remained "stable," but the emotional distance between them had increased. Anne continued to worry when Brent's job took him out of town during the day or he was late returning home. She still couldn't piece together how Brent—the man who loved her and had shared so much with her—could also be the man who had betrayed and hurt her so. She eventually stopped talking with Brent about her thoughts and feelings because these upset him. She found it increasingly difficult to let herself go when they were making love. Brent noticed her distance and interpreted it as Anne's efforts to punish him. When they returned to therapy, Brent continued to focus on Anne's mistrust and preoccupation with his affair as evidence that she needed to "erase" this from her thoughts. Her need to understand his affair more fully, and his insistence that they move on by not discussing it, created an impasse. Several months later Brent moved out, and eventually he and Anne divorced.

Is this outcome common? Unfortunately, yes. Is it inevitable? Thankfully, no. About 60–75% of couples remain married following discovery or disclosure of a partner's affair. Although some of these relationships continue to suffer lingering effects of the affair, other couples are able to use this crisis to identify changes they could make to restore emotional security and joy between them. Many relationships end up stronger, because the couple responded to the affair by working through the process of finding meaning described here and in the next few chapters.

Gail's affair came out of nowhere six months after the couple's youngest child left for college. She didn't blame Colin, her husband of 30 years. Colin was pleasant, diligent, and clearly loved Gail. But something was missing. When Gail was assigned responsibility for consulting with the manager of a competing firm about a possible merger, she and he "merged" in ways she had never anticipated. She felt like a college student again.

The affair was over in two months. At age 52, Gail wasn't about to throw away everything she had worked for over a brief fling. But she wasn't about to spend quiet evenings in front of the TV with Colin every night for the rest of her life either.

Gail had to come to grips with needs she had placed on hold for the past 15 years, but would be denied no longer. Colin had to grapple with being 7 years older than Gail and having less energy and more achy joints, as well as a wish to take life more slowly now that their youngsters had left. After weeks of shouting and tears from both, they agreed to arrange evenings out each week and weekends away each month—varying between slower-paced retreats and more action-filled ventures. Colin braved a visit to his doctor to get help for the sexual arousal problems he had struggled with on and off for the past several years. Gail pursued more frequent adventures with women from her office to add variety to her weekly routines.

They compromised, they persisted, and they moved on. It wasn't the perfect marriage—but it became better than it had been for each of them.

The goal of this chapter and the accompanying exercises is to help lay a good foundation for examining the affair by addressing:

- Whether some things are better left alone and not discussed.
- How to evaluate your readiness (and your partner's) to begin this next stage of recovery.
- How to proceed if your partner is reluctant or unwilling to join you in this process.

How Much Do We Need to Know?

As the lists of what you need to talk about in Chapter 2 demonstrate, the answer to this question is "a lot." An affair calls everything into question. And from the injured partner's perspective, beneath any unturned stone lurks another danger—the chance that whatever led to this affair could lead to another.

Because there's so much ground to cover, your attempts at understanding will probably feel jumbled or incomplete unless you find some organized way to explore. Each of the following chapters focuses on a different area or set of factors that may have increased the vulnerability of your relationship to an affair. These areas are introduced here to show you the types of questions you're going to be considering in more depth throughout Part II. You're probably already thinking about many of them, but seeing the full range will give you an idea of what you're in for so you can begin to determine whether you're ready for this work. It's important *not* to rush to conclusions at this point, so don't dwell on the questions. Just read them as an overview.

What Was Happening in Your Relationship

Affairs don't occur because of a bad marriage. There are plenty of troubled marriages that don't end up experiencing an affair, and there are also lots of affairs that occur even when participating partners report that they've been generally satisfied with their marriages and in love with their spouses. We'll never suggest that you blame your marriage for the affair. However, it's also important that both of you take a hard look at what was going on in your relationship that helped to make it more vulnerable or susceptible to an affair. This is the mission of Chapter 7.

As you examine your relationship and the ways in which it became vulnerable to an affair, it will be important to consider four general areas:

- **Levels and sources of conflict.** How effective have you and your partner been in managing disagreements and reaching decisions together? How frequent or intense were arguments between you? Were important differences between you ignored or avoided because your conversations seemed to go nowhere or led to blowups? What kinds of issues have been difficult to resolve? In what ways have unresolved differences led to resentment or to one or both of you pulling back?
- **Emotional connectedness.** How frequently did you and your partner share your important thoughts and feelings with each other? In what ways did you provide support during times of sadness or disappointment? How did you encourage and celebrate each other's achievements? What common values, beliefs, or goals promoted a sense of closeness between you? Would you each say the two of you have been best friends? In what ways did you begin to grow apart?
- **Physical intimacy.** How satisfied were you with your sexual relationship? Did each of you initiate lovemaking or suggest ways to keep the spark alive? Was sex something you could talk about openly? How did you manage times when one of you was less interested in or frustrated with

your sexual relationship? In what other ways did you pursue affection and physical closeness—kissing, snuggling, holding hands, or offering gentle touches during the day?

• **Relationship expectations.** Prior to the affair, how well did your marriage meet your initial expectations? In what ways were your own roles as a partner or parent frustrating or disappointing? Were responsibilities for your relationship or family life shared fairly? Were you and your partner each maintaining a healthy balance between maintaining your relationship and pursuing your own individual needs?

These are important issues in any marriage. Like most couples, you can probably identify some areas of your marriage that worked better or were more satisfying than other areas. The "rule" for exploring these questions is to talk respectfully but honestly with each other. And don't discount what's been good just because of the affair; acknowledge and celebrate your relationship's strengths while scrutinizing its weaknesses.

What Was Happening Around and Outside of Your Relationship

Maintaining a strong relationship requires hard work. That work becomes even more difficult when either (1) other people actively undermine your efforts to care for one another and remain faithful or (2) you fail to receive adequate support and encouragement for your relationship. Responding to the former will require you and your partner to reduce or eliminate these negative factors. Responding to the latter requires that you identify and seek out more support for your relationship. Both will be tackled in Chapter 8. Specifically, you'll need to address each of the following:

• **Intrusions and distractions.** What outside tasks, if any, pulled you away from devoting more time and energy to your relationship? Was either of you devoting too many hours to work? What other responsibilities did either of you have outside the home? How was your time consumed by other responsibilities *in* the home—such as your children, household chores, or other home projects? To what extent was relationship time redirected to other activities such as hobbies or recreation that you pursued separately? Having a healthy relationship also means developing yourself as an individual, so engaging in activities without your partner isn't wrong or bad. How well did you and your partner balance your focus on you as a couple versus you as individuals?

• **Stressors.** In what ways were you or your partner struggling with stressors from outside your relationship? For example—a change in your job, move to a new community, money problems, physical illness, concerns in your extended family, recent arrival of a newborn, or difficulties with one or more of your children? How much did these stressors draw you and your partner closer together, and in what ways did they push you farther apart?

• **Detractors and temptors.** How much time were you or your partner spending with individuals who place a low priority on relationships and fidelity? Were your friends single, recently divorced, or currently engaged in an affair? What aspects of your or your partner's life presented opportunity for an affair—such as frequent trips away from home, or extended time alone with someone at work or in the community? Does the nature of your work or activity outside the home put you in touch with other people who might be interested in an affair?

• **Supporters.** How much time were you and your partner spending with individuals or organizations that place a high priority on relationships and fidelity—either separately or together as a couple? How much did you seek out support and encouragement from these persons when you experienced distress or conflict in your relationship?

What the Participating Partner Brought to the Affair

As the injured party, you need to figure out how your partner had this affair—regardless of whatever else was going on between or around you. Viewing your partner only in negative ways—as fundamentally defective and without moral fiber—may fit with the hurt and anger you feel, but won't help to restore feelings of closeness or security. You need to be able to view your partner using a wide-angle lens—seeing strengths as well as shortcomings, virtues as well as flaws—to reach good decisions about how to move on.

As a participating partner, it's also important that you carefully examine what aspects of yourself contributed to your having an affair. *Most participating partners have an affair with mixed feelings, experience some level of guilt or sadness afterward, and describe some confusion about how they could have let themselves get involved in such a relationship.* So it's important that as the partner participating in the affair you ask, "What was going on with *me?*" Even if you don't ask that question of yourself, you already know that your partner will be asking this about you. "How could you have done this? What in the world were you thinking? Why were you willing to risk our marriage?" When you feel under attack, it's hard to respond to such questions and take a hard look at yourself because your partner may already see you in very negative ways. Or you might have tried to be open and honest, only to find that whatever you said wasn't accepted or was never enough. We hope the turmoil in your relationship has decreased enough that you can take more risk in confronting your own contributions. If this affair has brought unhappiness to you as well as to your partner, examining yourself, including your own personal needs or conflicts, will help you ensure that this doesn't happen to you again, whether you stay in this marriage or not. *Promising never to have another affair isn't enough.* You meant it when you made that vow the first time. Understanding how you got here and what you need to change will help you keep any new vows you make to yourself or someone else.

Chapter 9 aims to help you both gain this fuller understanding by examining the following areas:

- **Personal qualities increasing vulnerability to an affair.** In what ways did feelings of self-doubt about physical attractiveness, adequacy as a sexual partner, social or professional standing, or basic worth as a person increase the participating partner's susceptibility to an affair? Alternatively, did feelings of confidence, success, or other positive qualities put your partner at risk by making her especially attractive to others? Is your partner a naturally outgoing person who connects well with others? Do others confide easily in your partner, creating the likelihood of more intimate relationships? Did your partner fail to "keep up his guard" or set needed boundaries with other people because he didn't think an affair could happen to him?

- **Beliefs about affairs and commitment to your relationship.** What beliefs did your partner have about affairs prior to having one, and where did these beliefs come from? Did he or she hope for romance, play, passion, or excitement and see the affair as a way of gaining these qualities? Has your partner found it difficult to keep a promise, stick with a burdensome task, or resist temptations before? What kinds of commitments have been particularly difficult? What factors made it harder or easier to keep these? What would it take from your partner to commit to a difficult, lengthy process of working toward recovery from the affair?

- **Barriers to moving on.** What could be making it difficult for your partner to move on? If the affair is continuing, why won't your partner end it? If it's over, what's still getting in the way? How can your partner move from thoughts and feelings rooted in the past to creating a better future together?

What the Injured Partner Contributed to the Context for the Affair

Before you get into Chapter 10, remember that you didn't cause your partner to have an affair. When we encourage you to consider aspects of yourself that may relate to your partner's affair, we're not talking about your blame or responsibility. Instead, your aim in Chapter 10 should be to answer this question: "If my marriage became vulnerable to an affair because of conflict, emotional disconnection, outside commitments, or any other reason, could I have contributed to that vulnerability? What could I have done differently?" Your feelings of emotional security, in this or any future relationship, may continue to be influenced by feelings of vulnerability caused by the affair. You need to know that you've taken steps to address any way in which you may have contributed to your relationship's increased vulnerability so you'll feel better protected in the future.

As the participating partner, it's also important to read through Chapter 10 to understand both *why* and *how* you need to help your injured partner in this task. Only *you* know how your feelings about your relationship and your partner may have contributed to your affair. To answer the questions raised in that chapter, your partner will need information that you alone can share. Just as important as any information you may have will be your ability to encourage your partner through this process by making it emotionally safe.

Some of the areas you'll need to examine are similar to contributing factors we've identified for the participating partner; others are unique to the injured partner. All of them are addressed in Chapter 10.

- **Feelings about yourself.** Looking back, what kinds of feelings were you having about yourself prior to your partner's affair? How secure, attractive, or successful did you feel? How lonely, unhappy at home or at work, unsure of yourself, or frustrated with your life were you feeling? Consider how these feelings—either positive or negative—were expressed in your relationship. How far back do some of these feelings go? What were you needing from your partner or marriage? Reflect also on positive aspects of yourself that may have put your relationship at risk. For example, are you a generous or successful person on whom others place numerous demands and expectations, making it difficult for you to find time for your family?

• **Contributions to your marriage.** If conflict, emotional or sexual distance, or lack of play together contributed to your relationship's vulnerability, how might you have contributed to these? Independent of your partner, what could you have done differently to reduce problems or strengthen your marriage? If you never recognized prior to the affair some of the relationship problems you've now identified in looking back, how might you have been more vigilant? Your partner's affair may have happened despite a healthy, loving relationship between you; we don't want you to take responsibility for relationship problems that didn't actually exist. However, efforts to strengthen your marriage now will benefit from an honest self-appraisal by each of you.

• **Responses to personal injuries.** In what ways have you ever felt deeply disappointed or hurt in relationships prior to this one? How did you deal with those personal injuries then? How have you and your partner dealt with deep hurt between you in the past? How have your previous hurts or injuries—whether in earlier relationships or in this one—influenced your responses to this affair?

Taking It a Step at a Time

Each of these questions probably leads to others. The process of exploring all the factors that could have helped to create a context for an affair takes time and hard work. But in our experience, couples who pursue this second stage of recovery often end up addressing individual or relationship problems that have been present for years, as well as building on strengths that they've always had.

It's important that you work through these next chapters a step at a time. We can't tell you precisely what the right pace will be for you, because people and relationships vary. If you rush through this next stage too quickly, you won't examine some contributing factors closely or deeply enough; then you'll either (1) continue to feel uneasy or frustrated with lingering issues that haven't been addressed or (2) settle on an incomplete picture that leaves your relationship more vulnerable later on. But if you labor over each question too long or recycle endlessly over the same issues, you'll remain stuck and eventually one or both of you won't continue.

The process needs to be tailored to the emotional and time resources you can each commit, as well as to your ability to keep your interactions constructive. One approach is to set aside two to three times per week, for about 30 minutes on each occasion, to discuss what you've read or share your responses to an exercise. Each chapter has several parts, and discussions may benefit from your focusing solely on one part before moving on to the next. At the end of each interaction with your partner, try to agree on when you'll get together next and what you'll read or work on before then.

As best you can, be sure to spend just as much time together each week *not* discussing the affair but, instead, restoring positive ways of being together that you enjoyed in the past. You won't have either the hope or the emotional energy essential to getting through this next stage without caring for yourselves and your relationship.

Avoid getting stuck for too long on any one question. It's not only possible but likely that you and your partner will continue to have different perspectives on the affair—at least for a while. If you're getting hung up on an issue and can't reach some common understanding after two or three discussions, move on to the next section or next chapter. You can always come back to an earlier issue, and the work you've done between times may help you reconsider previous questions from a different perspective.

Are Some Things Better Left Not Discussed?

The goal is to help you both gain the information you need for eventually "settling things down" and "keeping things safe." Discussions that don't contribute to those two goals may not be examining the right questions or exploring these questions in the right way. But you can also get sidetracked onto some unproductive tangents. In particular, avoid these two kinds of discussions:

1. Getting into the gory, explicit details of what sexual behaviors did or didn't take place. More often than not, such information doesn't do much to improve a couple's own sexual relationship and only promotes

vivid images that can haunt the injured partner and make recovery more difficult.

2. Focusing on qualities of the third party that the participating partner found particularly attractive, especially qualities that the injured partner doesn't have or that the marriage currently lacks. Comparisons of a marriage partner with an affair partner are unfair because affair relationships differ tremendously from a marriage. Affair partners have the luxury of devoting their limited time and interactions to pleasing each other with relatively few distractions and burdens from the outside. You don't have to worry in an affair about paying for a new dishwasher, interacting with the other person's extended family, taking care of children together, or similar hassles. Put another way, the kinds of behaviors exchanged by persons in an affair aren't a good sampling of how they'd interact if they were married to each other. That's why *the majority of marriages that begin as affair relationships eventually end in divorce.*

Moreover, if you're the participating partner, there's a good possibility that some of the characteristics you found desirable in the other person or in the relationship with that person may have been present in your partner or marriage as well, but declined over time because of aspects of the marriage to which you contributed. Holding your partner solely responsible for whatever was lacking in the marriage or for how he may have started responding to your own behaviors just isn't realistic.

Finally, there may be other things about your partner that aren't fair to criticize. Your partner can't help getting older. She may not be responsible for health problems that get in the way of activities you used to enjoy or the stress brought on by children whom you helped to bring into your relationship. Or your partner may worry about the costs of flowers or dining out because the two of you are already struggling to make ends meet and have to be more accountable for your money in ways that persons in an affair don't.

In short, when examining factors that potentially caused your relationship to be more vulnerable to an affair, try to stay focused on what it would take to lower these risks. If things were missing from your marriage or you were looking for things from your partner that you didn't get, definitely discuss these factors. But don't set up such a discussion as a comparison between your partner and the person with whom you had an affair. Comparisons of that ilk usually just lead to more hurt and anger.

How Do We Know If We're Ready?

You may never feel *completely* ready to begin this next stage of recovery, and if you wait until you're each completely comfortable, pain-free, and immune to heated arguments, you'll probably never take this step. In our experience, many of the couples moving into this second stage of recovery do so with a certain amount of anxiety or mixed feelings. Pursuing this next stage doesn't involve being comfortable. Instead, it requires *understanding* what's going to be involved, *having the skills* vital to a successful process, and *being willing* to persist even when the process becomes difficult.

You and your partner need to understand what to expect and be as prepared as you can be. That's why we outlined general areas for you to examine and some of the specific questions to consider in each of these areas. However, you can't realistically anticipate every issue that will surface, what you'll learn, or how you're each going to respond to whatever you do discover. What's necessary is that you appreciate why this process is important, have a general idea of the kinds of issues and questions you'll be examining, and can envision how the understanding you'll achieve together can benefit each of you and potentially restore a secure relationship.

To be able to do this requires skills for (1) talking about your thoughts and feelings about this affair and (2) managing your feelings when your discussions become overheated and are no longer constructive (see Chapter 3). It also requires some ability to adopt each other's perspective. If you're not able to suspend your own thoughts and feelings long enough to even *hear* your partner's experience, you may not be ready to get what you should out of this stage. But even if so, start anyway. The only way you may develop this ability is with practice and determination.

Which leads to the last condition—*being willing*. In fact, you need to be not just willing but also determined and persistent. You should be prepared to hang in there even when the going gets tough. It will help if you support each other's commitment by acknowledging your partner's willingness to engage in this process, by having patience with each other when the process goes badly, by taking responsibility for your own contributions, and by making sure that even small steps forward are recognized and encouraged.

What If I'm Ready and Willing, but My Partner Isn't?

It's not unusual for one partner to be less eager to explore the context for the affair than the other. Like Brent, the husband described at the beginning of this chapter, participating partners are sometimes reluctant to engage in this process. They mostly just want to move on and put the affair behind them without dwelling on it, possibly because they don't feel as bewildered by the affair or as vulnerable to being hurt by a future affair, but also for all the other reasons discussed on pages 35–36 in Chapter 2.

Less frequently, injured partners may be reluctant to explore the affair, often because they're worried that if they push the issue too hard, the participating partner, who didn't want to talk about it anymore in the first place, may decide it's just not worth it and leave the marriage entirely. Such couples often reach an unspoken agreement not to talk about the affair again. As Anne discovered, however, such agreements can rarely be kept, because the injured partner's need to gain a fuller understanding is too compelling. Injured partners also sometimes feel unready for this exploration because they're still too angry to be able to collaborate or listen constructively or because they still feel traumatized and are seeking safety in emotional isolation. Some injured partners resist because it just feels too hurtful and frightening to take the next step. Sometimes this fear gradually diminishes on its own; other times it needs to be challenged directly by confronting the risks of *not* taking the next step.

Whether you're the injured partner or the participating partner, *if you're ready but your partner resists going through this process, you have a few options:*

- You can talk through your partner's reasons for the reluctance in an effort to move past this and then work together collaboratively.
- You can do most of the work by yourself, but then try to share the results of your efforts with your partner to invite a response.
- You can pursue the process completely separately from your partner and then use what you've learned to work at change by yourself—either for the sake of staying in this relationship or to be better informed about yourself and relationships generally if you decide to end this one.

Encouraging Your Partner to Join You

You may be able to influence your partner's decisions by talking about why this next stage is important to you, acknowledging your partner's reluctance, and exploring a process that could possibly work for both of you. What probably *won't* work are threats or coercion. Instead, try the following:

- *Discuss your concerns about not examining how the affair came about.* Talk about what you're afraid may happen if you don't explore the context of the affair more fully, or try writing a letter expressing these concerns. Ask your partner to read the first parts of this chapter and then request a 15-minute discussion about what this means to each of you. For example, as the injured partner, you might focus on the need for a fuller understanding as a way of feeling safer in the relationship. Or if you're the participating partner, you might express your concerns about not resolving problems in your relationship that potentially contributed to unhappiness for either one of you well before the affair.
- *Discuss potential advantages of doing this.* Talk about what you hope to come from this process for both of you. For example, how would you like your marriage to be six months from now, and how would working together help to bring these changes about?
- *Express your confidence in your ability to do this.* Talk about why you believe you're both ready and able to do this. Maybe you can point to progress you've made so far, or you could describe earlier times in your relationship when you were able to work together to address problems. What characteristics do you see in each of you that encourage you about being able to do this now?
- *Negotiate a process you each could commit to.* You may both believe in the importance of moving toward this next stage of recovery but have different ideas of just how to do this. What initial steps could you agree on—for example, each of you reading the next chapter over the next week and then getting together to work on the exercises? What alternative strategies might you consider if your initial efforts don't work as well as you'd like? Try to identify specific concerns or risks your partner anticipates and commit yourself to specific steps you're willing to take to reduce these concerns.

Sharing Your Efforts with Your Partner

For now, your partner may be willing to engage in this next stage only "partway." Maybe for now she won't read through the chapters and exercises with you, but she will have discussions with you based on your own reading. Admittedly, this won't work as well as if you work on this stage together, but *any* constructive work together is better than none, so try to find an initial compromise that will allow you to share your thoughts and feelings as you work through the next few chapters.

If you're the reluctant partner, please understand that encouraging your partner to share his efforts without your working on these issues as well may eventually fall short. Given what you've been through because of the affair, your relationship probably isn't going to recover fully until you're each convinced of your partner's commitment to doing whatever it takes to move forward.

Working Separately by Yourself

If your partner still won't participate in this next stage of recovery, it's important that you go ahead and do this work by yourself. Your partner may eventually recognize the importance of this work and may accept the challenge of exploring the context for the affair as well; if so, this may go better if you've already done this on your own and can contribute some of the understanding you've achieved. But even if your partner *never* joins you in this process, you'll be better off if you've done this for yourself.

If you're having difficulty sorting through your thoughts and feelings or you feel uncertain about whether your perspective on the affair is balanced or complete, input from a caring but objective outsider—a family member, a close friend, your clergyperson, or a professional counselor—may help. Be sure you review the guidelines in Chapter 4 for deciding whom to talk with about the affair, along with information about different kinds of helping professionals presented in Chapter 5.

Working through this next stage of recovery on your own isn't the best way of examining the context of the affair if the goal is for you and your partner to restore a trusting and intimate relationship. But if it's the only option you have, try to do this in a way that serves you best and get whatever additional help or support you need.

What's Next?

Working together in examining factors that may have contributed to the affair will probably lead to some uncomfortable or heated discussions, in part because you'll be getting into particularly sensitive or difficult areas. So review the guidelines in Chapter 3 for how to talk with each other about feelings, solve problems, and reach decisions together and for using constructive time-outs to defuse heated arguments. Above all, work hard at understanding each other's perspectives on how this affair came about.

If your partner hasn't yet read this chapter, encourage your partner to read it and request 15 to 20 minutes to discuss both of your reactions. Don't try to use this time to explore specific factors that contributed to the affair. Instead, use the time to discuss the *process* (not factors that may have contributed to the affair) and to reach a decision about how to move forward through this next stage. Whether together or separately on your own, work through the exercises that follow. Then continue working through the remaining chapters that examine different areas of potential contributing factors to the affair.

Remember to hang in there! You probably already recognize that this next stage of work will be difficult. But also remember that it's critical.

———————————— Exercises ————————————

To undertake the important but difficult process of exploring why the affair came about, it's essential that you have clear in your own mind (1) what you hope to get from the process and (2) what might make it hard for you. The exercises in this chapter are intended to focus on these two issues.

It's best if you and your partner first complete the exercises for each chapter in Part II separately, write down your individual responses, and then schedule a time to exchange your responses with each other and discuss them before going on to the next chapter. Remember to limit your discussions to 30 minutes at any given time and then schedule additional discussions as needed to work through your respective responses. Follow the communication guidelines outlined in Chapter 3. If your conversations get too heated, take a break and try again later when you're both feeling calmer. If your partner isn't working through this book with you, complete the exercises on your own and then see whether your partner might be willing to talk with you for 15 to 30 minutes to discuss the issues addressed in these exercises. If your partner won't join you in exploring the issues raised in these exercises, use them for yourself to come to a fuller understanding of how the affair came about.

EXERCISE 6.1.
IDENTIFYING WHAT YOU HOPE TO GAIN FROM THIS PROCESS

Keeping in mind what you want to gain from this process can help to keep you motivated when the going gets tough. In addition, knowing what you hope to gain can help to guide you through the process. *"If I want to achieve this goal, here's what I need to do or focus on."*

Decide what you hope to gain from exploring the affair and trying to understand why it happened. For example, as the injured partner you might experience:

"Mainly, I feel so confused that I need to understand why this happened because I can't make any sense of my life or our relationship right now."

Or

"Until I know why this happened, I can't decide whether to stay in this relationship. If I know why it happened, maybe I'll know if it's likely to happen again or how we need to change things."

Or as the participating partner you might think:

"I never thought I'd do this. It's not consistent with my values. I need to understand better how this happened to know whether my partner and I can make the changes we need to for our relationship to work."

Write down at least two things you hope to gain by exploring why the affair occurred. Then share these objectives with your partner and discuss why you need to understand what happened and how you believe it will benefit each of you. As you work through the remaining chapters in this section of the book, look back occasionally at what you've written down here. Make sure you're exploring the affair in a way that addresses what you hope to learn and why you're doing this.

EXERCISE 6.2.
IDENTIFYING POTENTIAL HAZARDS AND HOW YOU'LL HANDLE THEM

Exploring the full range of factors that could have contributed to the affair can be difficult for both partners. The reasons for this vary from one person to the next. Why might this be hard for you? For example, are there particular aspects of your relationship or yourself that you find difficult to discuss? Are there particular patterns of talking with your partner that seem to get in the way? Identifying potential hazards that could make it more difficult to explore how the affair came about can help you develop strategies for overcoming those barriers.

Identify potential hazards that could make it harder for you to explore factors that made your marriage vulnerable to an affair. There may be things about you that you don't want to confront. For example:

"I think I was a fool not to see what was going on. Focusing on that will just make me feel worse about myself."

Or

"I'm afraid to hear about how I wasn't a good lover or fell short as a partner in other ways."

Or you might be fearful of what you'll learn about your partner:

"I'm worried I might realize that I'm not married to the person I thought was so wonderful and right for me. If I come to believe that, I might have to end the relationship."

You might also fear what you'll see about your relationship:

"I'm really scared I'll find out that our marriage was a failure all along and I was just denying it—or that we really can't make it work."

Alternatively, you might be worried about what will happen between you and your partner if you discuss the affair.

"If I force my partner to talk about it, I'm afraid she'll leave for good."

Or

"Each time we try to talk about it, we have horrible screaming matches. I can't take it anymore, and at times I'm afraid things might get violent."

Outline specific steps that you or your partner can take to address these concerns. For example:

"For now, I'm just going to be honest and see what I can learn, even if it means recognizing some things about me, my partner, or our relationship that I don't like. I'll continue to remind myself that just because we have problems or flaws, that doesn't mean things are hopeless."

Or

"To keep things manageable when we discuss the affair, we'll go over our communication guidelines first. We'll agree what to do if things become too heated (for example, take a time-out), and we'll set a limit on how long to talk so we don't get too tired to stay focused and constructive."

As you work through the upcoming chapters, review what you've listed as your concerns and how you're managing them. Make sure you remain aware of these hazards and that you're following your planned strategies. If new concerns arise along the way, add them to your list along with specific strategies for handling them.

>>>

7

Was My Marriage to Blame?

Kathy and Paul had "the perfect marriage." In each other they had found the person they had always dreamed of marrying. In Paul, Kathy found a man who was strong, responsible, and had a clear vision of the future. And in Kathy, Paul found a woman who brought warmth and passion to a life that had seemed cold and dreary. The first few years of their marriage were happy and satisfying. They started a successful business together, and their respective families boasted with pride about their accomplishments. They were invited to join exclusive social groups in the community. They had two new cars fully paid for and a nice new home. Life was good.

Several years into their marriage, they decided it was time to begin a family of their own. Kathy turned managing their business over to Paul while she stayed home to care for their two sons who arrived over the next three years. Pleased at first with these decisions, neither was prepared for their new roles.

Kathy missed her interactions with business colleagues. She had few friends of her own and turned increasingly to Paul for comfort and relief from the youngsters when he came home in the evenings. The more she needed Paul, however, the less available he appeared to be. His hours at work grew longer, and his patience at home seemed to grow shorter. When she tried to tell Paul how lonely or un-supported she felt, he responded with how unappreciated he felt for his efforts to support the family financially. Kathy felt increasingly desperate and alone.

Paul struggled too. This wasn't what he had expected fatherhood to feel like. The boys seemed attached to Kathy, not to him. He was uncomfortable holding them when they cried; he felt impatient when they got into things they shouldn't or constantly demanded his attention. Kathy couldn't appreciate his difficulties with the boys and frequently seemed angry at him for reasons he didn't understand. Paul felt increasingly inadequate both as a husband and as a father.

When their sons reached two and three years of age, Kathy placed them in day care two afternoons each week so that she could take a business class at their community college. There she found other men and women her age who were juggling multiple challenges of work, family, and school. Many had concerns and interests similar to hers. One in particular, Ben, was particularly friendly to Kathy and seemed especially understanding. Ben and Kathy worked on a class presentation together but found themselves spending increasing amounts of time talking about Kathy's frustrations at home. Ben was divorced, and Kathy found herself admiring his devotion to his daughter from that marriage. Increasingly Kathy felt herself drawn to Ben, which made her feel so disloyal to Paul that she tried hard to connect with him when he got home from work. But Paul was frequently too tired to talk, or fell asleep as soon as they went to bed. More and more, their evenings ended in arguments.

Over the next month, Ben made it clear how strongly he was drawn to Kathy. He empathized with her loneliness, and both felt an increasing emotional and physical attraction. Brief interactions in class were often followed by long, intimate conversations by phone and by brief but frequent contact by cell phone or instant-messaging on the computer throughout the day. Eventually, following a particularly difficult week with Paul when they had argued almost constantly and slept in separate rooms, Kathy visited Ben at his apartment. She felt abandoned by Paul and despaired of his ever being able to understand her. She knew having an affair would be wrong, but her longing to be held and comforted overcame her. She and Ben ended up in bed together that afternoon, then twice more in the following week.

Over the next two months Kathy saw Ben whenever she could, but wrestled with guilt and confusion about the dual life she was leading. She wasn't sure she wanted to stay married to Paul, but she eventually concluded that she couldn't continue her affair. She broke off her relationship with Ben, but two weeks later disclosed her affair to Paul and asked that they try living separately for a while to give them space to reach a decision about their marriage. Both of them felt hurt, angry, and confused. Paul felt devastated and utterly betrayed by Kathy; nothing he had done deserved this. But he also didn't want to end their marriage. He didn't want to move out, but reluctantly agreed when the next week seemed to be one endless hurtful argument.

Two weeks after Paul moved out, he and Kathy agreed they needed help to reach a decision about what to do next. In couple therapy they were able to reach some short-term decisions about how to interact with each other and around their children. Once they got through their initial crisis, they began to consider all that had gone wrong. How did this happen? Not very long ago they had had the perfect marriage. How did it come tumbling apart?

When your partner has had an affair, you'll probably eventually ask yourself, "Was my marriage to blame?" As we've said before, the answer is no. Responsibility rests with the person who chose to have an affair. But as we've also said before, you *should* consider how your marriage became vulnerable to an affair. Were important qualities missing? Were there ways you two could have made your relationship stronger? If you look back, you may be able to identify several aspects of your relationship that weren't as satisfying as either one of you might have liked. Keep in mind, though, that the goal isn't to lay blame; it's to figure out how you could make your marriage more secure now.

In the process, you might gain a better perspective on other factors that contributed to the affair. Right now, for example, your mind may be reeling with accusations about your partner: he had the affair because he's unloving, can't commit, or can't be trusted. You're right to want to know how your partner could have done such a hurtful thing. But remember that this is the same person you fell in love with, married, and expected to spend the rest of your life with. To make sense of how this man you've loved could have done such a hurtful thing, it's important to consider how your relationship contributed to the context within which he decided to have an affair.

Participating partners need to gain the same insight. Few, if any, made a vow of commitment while *aspiring* to infidelity. Many that we've counseled, in fact, have confessed to being bewildered by how they could have ended up on this path. To make sense of their own behavior, participating partners as well as injured partners need to examine not only aspects of themselves individually but also contributing risk factors outside themselves, including the relationship itself.

In this chapter we'll offer a process for doing that, first encouraging you to examine various aspects of your relationship in the three to four months prior to the beginning of the affair. Then we'll help you look at your marriage from a broader perspective—including initial sources of attraction and personal styles of relating that may have influenced how you and your partner have interacted from early in your relationship. Finally, we'll help you address one of the most important questions you'll face: *Given everything you and your partner can learn about potential vulnerabilities in your marriage, what would it take to make your relationship more secure now?*

As you go through this chapter, remember that you're looking at only one part of the puzzle. Try to avoid settling on any one conclusion about how this affair came about too early in this process. Usually many different factors contributed to how an affair initially came about and how it continued or ended. Premature conclusions based on a limited view of how the affair occurred can get in the way of examining the bigger picture. For now, just as in putting together a large jigsaw puzzle, first try to get all the pieces out on the table. Initially it may be clear how some of the pieces fit together or form a pattern, but the role that other pieces play may elude you at first. You can wait to figure out some of that until later, after you work through Chapters 8 to 10, which help you examine other aspects of your life as a couple and as individuals.

In addition, try to distinguish among different time periods in your relationship—for example, during courtship, the first few years of marriage, and the last few years. Try not to let your struggles since the affair determine how you view your relationship in earlier years. It's not uncommon for relationships to go through both good and not-so-good periods. Understanding both sides can help you assess the potential for your marriage when it's at its best and begin to identify factors that have contributed or still contribute to relationship difficulties.

What Was Our Marriage Like before the Affair?

The following questions address a variety of issues that can expose relationships to distress and may have made your relationship more vulnerable. These questions don't cover all possible concerns, but can help to get you started in this process.

How Well Did We Deal with Differences?

One of the most common complaints among distressed couples involves difficulties in managing conflict. The specific form that such conflict takes can vary a great deal. For some couples, differences are rarely acknowledged or openly discussed; however, either partner may feel frustrated or resentful when issues important to that person aren't recognized or resolved. Such couples often display a "demand/withdraw" pattern in which one partner repeatedly expresses concerns or complaints, while the other partner withdraws from the discussion or refuses to engage in the conflict. For other couples, even minor differences frequently escalate into major arguments; a pattern of intense conflict with few agreements leads to a backlog of unresolved differences that drives partners apart emotionally and physically. Still other couples describe a pattern of frequent bickering that erodes their sense of closeness or liking for one another; tensions may occasionally erupt into major conflicts, but more often they're evident from minor but frequent skirmishes with no predictable pattern.

Any one of these patterns for dealing with differences contributes to a couple's distress and may increase a marriage's vulnerability to an affair. To examine how well you and your partner dealt with differences between you before the affair, consider levels and sources of conflict as well as strategies for managing them. We'll raise initial questions for you to consider here. Then, in Exercise 7.1, we'll ask you to pull together your answers to develop a clearer picture of how you two have managed conflict and how you could do it more effectively in the future.

Levels of Conflict

It's not that you two disagree—virtually all couples have disagreements—but how you manage the differences that matters. The frequency, intensity, and duration of conflicts can increase your relationship's vulnerability to an affair.

How *often* did you and your partner battle in the few months before the affair? Had arguments become more common, perhaps reflecting a growing frustration or impatience either of you felt with your relationship? Or had arguments become less frequent, perhaps because one of you had given up on resolving differences over important issues?

How *intense* were the conflicts? Did they typically involve minor bickering or major arguments that escalated out of proportion? Did they lead either one of you to threaten or consider divorce?

How *long* did your arguments last—a few minutes, a few hours, or a few days? Following a disagreement, how long did it typically take you to reconnect either by resolving the difference or by accepting it and moving on? Did you and your partner frequently have different "recovery times"?

Sources of Conflict

Ask someone what couples most frequently argue about, and common answers include sex, money, children, and in-laws. Many times, however, the picture is somewhat more complicated. Conflicts about children, for example, may involve differences in fundamental values, expectations regarding partners' respective child rearing responsibilities, beliefs about best methods of discipline, or underlying struggles for control. If you and your partner have trouble pinpointing the primary sources of conflict in your relationship or disagree on what might help to eliminate or reduce the conflict, step back and ask yourself, "What else might be going on here that we're not recognizing?"

>>> **Common sources of relationship conflict include:**
- **Specific areas of interaction.**
- **Marriage and family boundaries.**
- **Shared resources.**
- **Opportunities and responsibilities.**
- **Differences in preferences or values.**
- **Differences in personal style.**

As you think about each of these areas, use the questions below to begin thinking about strengths in your relationship as well as problems.

Conflicts in Specific Areas of Interaction

Consider where you and your partner have experienced frequent or intense conflict—for example, about finances, the children, your sexual relationship, how to spend your leisure time, or how to divide responsibilities in the home. Try to prioritize or rank order these into the "hottest" two or three conflict areas. How have conflicts in these areas changed over the years? Also try to identify one or two times when you managed differences in these areas with less conflict. What did you and your partner do differently at those times that seemed to work better? This might help you find ways to manage differences more effectively in the future.

Conflicts Related to Marriage and Family Boundaries

If you worked through Chapters 2 and 3, you've already set some boundaries to define various interactions. Now think about how boundaries, or a lack thereof, may have contributed to conflicts in the past. Do you and your partner agree on how much time to spend either separately or together with your children, friends, or respective families? What kinds of communication or other activities do you restrict to yourselves only—for example, discussions of your physical intimacy?

Conflicts Related to Shared Resources

Some couples have difficulty defining "yours, mine, or ours" in different areas, from money and material objects to time and physical space in the home. Sometimes these conflicts result from the complexity of the situation itself—for example, how to deal with an inheritance intended for the college education of children in a blended family in which different children have different sets of extended families with very different financial assets. Other conflicts seem trivial but can trigger equally strong feelings—such as how to divide the space in a cramped clothes closet. What strategies did you and your partner use to promote feelings of fairness for both of you?

Conflicts Related to Opportunities and Responsibilities

Partners sometimes struggle with how to balance opportunities and responsibilities, both in their own lives and in their relationship. For example, pursuing a career outside the home may be viewed by one partner as an opportunity but by the other as a responsibility to provide financially for the family. When couples maintain a "team identity," each partner can contribute in different ways and at different times to the marriage in ways that feel fair and mutually encouraging. In what ways have you and your partner struggled to maintain a "team identity" in your own relationship?

Conflicts Related to Different Preferences and Values

Relationship conflict can result from differences in preferences or core values—and distinguishing between these is important. Preferences are akin to likes and dislikes, and differences here can often be tolerated or negotiated to find a middle ground. Differences in core values are more difficult to resolve. What happens when one partner believes deeply in the importance of saving for the future while the other believes just as strongly in living each day to the fullest because tomorrow may never come? Though that kind of value divergence can be tough to deal with, a bigger problem for some couples is that they label almost everything as a core value and nothing as a mere preference. When too many differences are framed as critical issues involving core values, partners can find themselves deeply stuck in opposing views and unwilling to budge toward a middle position. How often in the past have you and your partner found yourselves stuck in opposing positions? Looking back, how often did differences in preferences get mishandled as though they involved conflicting core values?

Conflicts Related to Differences in Personal Style

Considerable research has been conducted to determine whether in relationships "opposites attract" or "birds of a feather flock together." The conflicting evidence suggests that both occur and that what may matter most is the extent to which partners build on their respective strengths and differences. For example, relationships won't work well if both partners always insist on being in charge or if each consistently waits for the other to take the lead; instead, they'll work better when partners take turns or identify respective areas of expertise. To what extent have conflicts between you and your partner resulted from differences around such issues as liking to be in charge, a desire for time together versus time to be alone, or the wish to discuss feelings versus solving problems? Instead of undermining your marriage, how could you use such differences to strengthen it?

Ron and Elaine argued constantly about how to discipline their two young children. Ron's parents had been stern and punitive, and he was determined to have a closer and more relaxed relationship with his own children. Elaine grew up in a family torn apart by her older

165

brother's rebellious behavior and various legal problems, and she vowed that as a parent she would set firm limits from the very beginning. The stricter Elaine was with their children, the more Ron refused to participate in the rules and consequences she insisted on. Eventually they recognized their increasing polarization and began to work toward some middle ground they could each live with.

Difficulties in Managing Conflict

Because some level of conflict is inevitable in intimate relationships, couples need strategies for identifying differences, preventing conflicts from escalating into destructive arguments, and reaching decisions together in a way that resolves differences or makes them more tolerable.

>>> **Ineffective strategies for managing conflict may stem from:**
  - **Under- or overcontrol of feelings.**
  - **Differences in emotional and cognitive style.**
  - **Differences in timing.**
  - **Efforts to win.**

Under- or Overcontrol of Emotions

Relationships can suffer when the "temperature" of a couple's conflicts strays too far from moderate. Some couples run "too hot." Every disagreement, frustration, or disappointment—no matter how small—demands discussion about "what's wrong" and ignores "what's right" in the relationship. By contrast, some relationships run "too cold." Partners try to achieve comfort and safety by avoiding difficult but important discussions. Both undercontrol of conflict (running "hot") and overcontrol (running "cold") can put a relationship at risk. Before the affair, how much balance did you achieve in managing conflict, discussing important relationship issues but letting go of minor irritations or annoyances?

Differences in Emotional and Cognitive Style

Much has been written about how men and women differ in approaching conflict. There's some evidence that women are brought up to discuss feelings as a way of promoting closeness, whereas men are often encouraged to treat conflicts as problems to be solved through intellectual analysis. When one partner seeks to reduce conflict by talking about feelings and the other responds by adopting an analytical problem-solving style, both can feel frustrated and misunderstood. Because neither approach is inherently better than the other, it's important for partners to understand differences in their styles and learn how to accommodate both when dealing with relationship conflicts. Have you and your partner ever seemed "out of sync" when discussing differences? Has either of you viewed the other as too emotional or too detached?

Differences in Timing

Some people feel a strong need to resolve tensions right away, while others need time apart to gain perspective and control over their feelings. When one partner seeks immediate resolution and the other needs time to reach emotional equilibrium or to deal with hurt feelings separately, efforts to resolve conflict together may not be productive. To what extent have you and your partner experienced different preferences in this area?

Efforts to Win

When efforts to resolve differences have less to do with collaboration and more to do with who's "right," more deserving of an apology, or will make the greater concession or go the extra distance in restoring peace, the relationship ends up losing. *Neither partner can win an argument without the other losing.* Strategies for resolving conflict work best in relationships when both partners shift from a focus on what *they* want to a focus on what their *marriage* needs. How often have efforts to resolve conflicts gotten stuck because they felt like a "win–lose" struggle? What would it take from *you* to promote a stronger sense of teamwork and collaboration?

> Both Sharon and Randy acknowledged being "strong willed." At work their persistence proved an asset, but at home they repeatedly ended up at odds with each other. When dealing with differences of opinion, Randy tended to become heated but would then cool down, apologize, and look for common ground. Sharon was uncomfortable with Randy's intensity and sometimes felt wounded by his comments; she continued to feel hurt long after Randy had already cooled down, and wasn't yet ready to resume discussion—a response that Randy viewed as unforgiving and punitive. Their discussions improved when

Randy exercised better control over how he expressed his opinions and when Sharon learned to tolerate some of her own discomfort with conflict.

Reducing the frequency and intensity of negative exchanges between you and your partner, and finding more effective ways to reach agreement on important issues, may provide a critical foundation for increasing your emotional or physical connection—topics we'll help you consider next.

How Emotionally Connected Did We Feel?

Most likely you and your partner weren't initially drawn to each other because of your ability to manage conflict. Instead, you were probably attracted to each other because you enjoyed each other's company. There was something about being with your partner that simply felt good. It may be because you shared similar interests and had fun together. Or perhaps you found your partner easy to talk with and able to understand your feelings. Perhaps your partner was especially supportive through a difficult time. Any one of these experiences helps to promote a feeling of being emotionally connected.

Partners can feel emotionally disconnected even when they're not experiencing conflict. In considering how your marriage became vulnerable to an affair, it's important to examine how well you and your partner worked together to promote feelings of emotional connection and closeness. Below we describe a variety of ways that couples sometimes use to promote closeness and intimacy in their relationships.

Sharing Experiences

Partners feel closer to each other when they arrange times to work side by side for the sole purpose of spending time together. For example, some couples make it a point to prepare meals or work in the yard together; others read stories to their children or run errands together. Happily married partners also make an effort to talk with each other about everyday experiences; discussions about ordinary or routine events convey a desire to share their lives even when apart.

On a deeper level, couples often feel most emotionally connected when one partner shares feelings of hurt or disappointment and the other listens in a caring and supportive way. Partners' abilities to share deep feelings, to have these feelings heard and understood, and to experience a tender caring for each other form the most important part of an intimate relationship. In thinking about your own relationship, how well did both you and your partner demonstrate your interest and concern for each other before the affair? Did you invite each other to share your deepest thoughts and feelings, and did you genuinely listen to each other?

Ways of becoming emotionally disconnected include:

- Not working together as a team to accomplish common tasks.
- Difficulty in sharing emotional experiences or feeling understood.
- Not sharing visions or dreams for the future.
- Not setting aside enough time to play together.

Sharing Visions

Partners feel emotionally connected when they share a common vision. The vision may be as simple as how to plan new landscaping in the yard. It may be as distant as where they want to retire in 30 years. Or it may be as complicated as how to live a spiritual or meaningful life as a couple and a family.

It's easy for couples to lose a sense of shared vision. We've listened to many couples describe how earlier in their courtship they used to sit for hours talking about their visions of how their family life would be: how many children to have and what to name them, what kind of dog to have, the design for the home they'd build out in the country, or places they'd travel to together. But years later the experience of sharing visions somehow got lost. Sometimes their dreams suffered under the weight of current disappointments, or the reality of today's demands offered little opportunity for dreaming about tomorrow.

Sharing a vision for the future can be as important as sharing feelings from today's events. Both can be deeply personal and intimate experiences. Right now, the future of your relationship may feel too uncertain to experience a shared vision. But try to recall the three to four months prior to the affair. How often did you and your partner share dreams for your future together?

Sharing Play

Sharing laughter, playing games, pursuing common activities, and exercising or simply relaxing together are some of the ways that partners reconnect. Research shows that couples who spend significant amounts of time together in common activities other than work also report more satisfaction with their relationship. Stated simply, couples who play together are more likely to stay together.

There are two general kinds of activities that couples use for reconnecting—each with their respective advantages. Engaging in "parallel" activities such as watching a movie, reading quietly in the same room, or attending an event together can be a way of sharing time and space when tensions between partners may make it more difficult to interact without getting into conflict or hurtful discussions. By contrast, "joint" activities such as preparing a romantic dinner together, going for a leisurely stroll, or pursuing a hobby together often work best when tensions between partners are fewer or can be put aside.

Some couples allow their playtime to suffer in response to such demands as child rearing, responsibilities at work, or commitments to their church or community. Often those who are first to take responsibility for others forget to set aside a portion of their time for caring for their own marriages. This oversight can erode a couple's sense of closeness. Play with one's partner restores a sense of couple identity.

Before the affair, how well did the two of you preserve separate time for yourselves to play together? When setting aside time for play, were you careful not to allow discussions about relationship problems to intrude? When previous ways of being together were no longer possible or lost their appeal, did you develop new ways of connecting through leisure time together?

How Physically Intimate Were We?

Nonsexual Intimacy

Just like emotional closeness, physical intimacy occurs on different levels. For many couples, touching and holding one another are just as important as sexual intimacy. In considering the quality of physical intimacy in your marriage prior to the affair, it may be useful to think first about physical closeness other than sexual exchanges. How often did you touch one another in nonsexual ways? For example, did you say good-bye or greet one another with a hug or kiss? How often did you hold hands when sitting together at a movie or ball game? Did you offer gentle or reassuring touches as you passed each other in the hallway or kitchen? Did you touch or hold each other in bed when not making love?

Individuals vary in how comfortable they are with physical touch and how much they desire touching in nonsexual ways. For example, it's not uncommon for women to be comfortable with and to desire nonsexual touching more than their husbands—although we've worked with many couples in whom this difference was reversed. Often differences in comfort with physical touch relate to how much physical affection was expressed in individuals' homes as they were growing up.

How important is it to you and your partner to be physically close in nonsexual ways? How do you each express your need for such closeness or respond to your partner's needs? For example, how regularly do you touch, hold hands, or exchange hugs? If you and your partner are different in this regard, how have you tried to find some middle ground? How physically affectionate were you around the time of the affair?

Sexual Intimacy

For most couples, sexual intimacy is closely tied to how emotionally connected the partners feel—with sexual intimacy occurring more often when partners feel emotionally close, or emotional closeness following from sexual intimacy, or both. When sexual intimacy declines or breaks down, partners' responses can range from hurt or disappointment to confusion or relief. Research shows that partners' satisfaction with their sexual relationship is strongly related to their overall satisfaction with their marriage.

Ways of becoming physically disconnected include:

- Insufficient touches, hugs, or other nonsexual forms of physical closeness.
- Differences in levels of sexual desire.
- Low frequency of lovemaking.
- Dissatisfaction with the quality of sexual intimacy.
- Difficulties in talking about sex.
- Barriers to sexual intimacy.

If sexual intimacy was a concern in your marriage, it's important to explore how this could have contributed to your vulnerability to an affair.

> Josh enjoyed sex with Wenona just about any time she was agreeable, which was once or twice a week—not bad, he thought, but not as often as he'd like. Wenona enjoyed sex with Josh when she wasn't stressed from work or from dealing with the children, but preferred relaxed and longer lovemaking—even if less often—to the frequent but sometimes rushed sex that Josh seemed comfortable with. Wenona didn't like disappointing Josh, and similarly he didn't like the idea of pressuring her. After a while they both found it easier to avoid dealing with differences around sex, and their lovemaking became less and less frequent. Neither felt happy about the situation, but they just couldn't seem to find ways of discussing it to make it better.

Differences in Sexual Desire and Low Frequency of Lovemaking

It's not unusual for partners to differ somewhat in their overall desire for sexual intimacy, or to differ in their sexual desire at any given time. About 15% of men and 25% of women report that their disinterest in sex is a problem for them or their relationship. Sexual intimacy is most likely to occur when both partners view lovemaking as an important part of their relationship, feel free to express their sexual desire, and assume some share of responsibility for initiating and responding to requests for lovemaking. Feelings of guilt, pressure, or blame detract from enjoyment of sexual exchanges. So do feelings of hurt, resentment, or overall unhappiness with the marriage.

Strongly related to low sexual desire in one or both partners is low frequency of sex. Although couples vary widely in how often they make love, a *common* range is two to three times per week to once every one to two weeks. Couples in their 20s tend to have intercourse more frequently than couples in their 50s. When sex occurs less often than once or twice a month, partners can begin to feel self-conscious or anxious about their sexual intimacy. This sometimes triggers a pattern of avoiding physical touch, hugs, or passionate kissing that frequently led to lovemaking in the past. This pattern of sexual avoidance is surprisingly common, with roughly one in five couples being sexual less than 10 times per year.

How have you and your partner handled occasions when one of you wanted to make love but the other preferred not to at that time? Did you both initiate lovemaking on different occasions? Have there been times in the past year or so when you and your partner went for several weeks or longer without being sexually intimate? Was the frequency of your lovemaking in the past six months significantly changed from earlier in your marriage? If so, did either of you express concern about this, and how did the other respond?

Dissatisfaction with the Quality of Sexual Intimacy

You and your partner may vary in what you find to be sexually arousing. For some people, the quality of lovemaking depends heavily on the level of romance—including soft music, candles, and nonsexual intimacy beforehand. For others, sexual intimacy is heightened by the experience of mutual physical passion—including the sheer intensity of movements, noisemaking, and raw sexual release. Some people enjoy sex most when they've been able to anticipate lovemaking throughout the day, using touches or glances as reminders of the intent to be sexual later that evening; others enjoy sex most when it's unplanned and spontaneous. Partners don't always agree on what they find sexually exciting or even comfortable.

Couples sometimes struggle under the pressure to achieve "great sex" every time they're sexually intimate. A more realistic expectation is that for many couples about 40–50% of sexual experiences will be very good for both partners; 20–25% are very good for one partner and fine for the other. About 20–25% of sexual exchanges are acceptable but not remarkable, and the remaining 10–15% are mediocre or unsatisfying. Failure to recognize this variety in sexual experiences within the same relationship can lead either partner to feel unnecessary disappointment, frustration, guilt, or resentment. Prior to the affair, did either or both of you experience dissatisfaction with the quality of your lovemaking?

Difficulties in Talking about Sex

You might experience difficulties in talking about your sexual relationship for many different reasons. For example, you might have difficulty in identifying or expressing feelings about lovemaking, or your partner may have difficulty in listening or responding to these feelings in a supportive way. Alternatively, your respective feelings and preferences may be very clear to both of you, but you're unable to reach decisions about how to resolve your differences or pursue mutual wants and needs effectively. Some couples are able to communicate effectively about anything *except* sex. For example, complaints about the sexual relationship may become part of a larger "laundry list" of complaints that get voiced during arguments over other issues. Or discussions about sexual difficulties may be initiated by one partner without warning (for example, while preparing dinner together), or they may occur primarily in bed, when one partner is feeling particularly frustrated.

Have you and your partner had difficulties talking about aspects of your own sexual relationship—for example, about how often to make love or about your respective likes and dislikes? Did you arrange for times to discuss your sexual relationship that felt less threatening or antagonistic to both? When you discovered differences, how did you go about finding compromises? How would you need to change your own role in discussions about your sexual relationship for these to go better?

Barriers to Sexual Intimacy

Even if you and your partner both have healthy sexual drives and similar sexual preferences, other factors can serve as barriers to sexual intimacy. One of the most common barriers that couples describe involves time pressures resulting from work and child rearing. Too often in the face of other demands, attending to the sexual relationship can seem like a luxury rather than a critical part of partners' staying connected. Another common barrier to sexual intimacy involves issues of physical and emotional health. Some people don't enjoy having sex if they're struggling with allergies, back pain, or physical fatigue—while others' sexuality seems unaffected by such concerns. Pregnancy and the first few months following childbirth often disrupt sexual intimacy—particularly if the couple's sexual exchanges prior to pregnancy primarily involved intercourse. Sexual desire, arousal, and performance can also be affected by emotional factors such as anxiety or depression—as well as by medications commonly used to treat these conditions.

Perhaps you or your partner struggle with specific sexual difficulties. If so, you're not alone. Common problems for men include difficulties in achieving or maintaining an erection, reaching climax too quickly, or difficulty in having an orgasm after extended stimulation. For women, common problems include pain during intercourse, difficulty in becoming aroused or lubricated despite having sexual desire, or difficulties in achieving orgasm. Almost half of women and about a third of men may experience one of these specific sexual problems at some time or another. Interestingly, specific sexual problems are often unrelated to sexual satisfaction or overall marital happiness. It's only when these problems contribute to additional feelings such as not being desired or cared for that couples experience higher risk for becoming emotionally and physically disconnected.

What barriers to sexual intimacy have you and your partner experienced? Knowing what you know now, how could you reduce these obstacles to sexual intimacy in your marriage? Exercise 7.2 is designed to help you use what you've learned here to understand how difficulties in emotional or physical connection may have made your relationship more vulnerable to an affair, and to guide you in considering what it would require to increase intimacy.

Were We Ever a Healthy Couple?

In the initial chaos following an affair, it's sometimes possible to lose a broader view of the marriage from a long-term perspective. As an injured partner, it may be difficult to recall earlier times when you were confident in the love and commitment you each brought to your marriage because right now you feel deeply hurt. Or you may now view those earlier confident feelings with suspicion, perhaps doubting your judgment or questioning how truthful your partner has ever been with you. As a participating partner, it may be difficult to focus on what you've valued most in your marriage because this seems at such odds with your decision to have an affair. "How could I have done this but still believe our getting married was the right decision?"

In evaluating whether you can make this marriage work again—and whether you even want to—you need to consider not only what was happening in the few months leading up to the affair, but also the broader picture of your marriage from the very beginning. What were the good reasons for marrying your partner? What have been your most worthwhile times together? It may also be true that there have been some important vulnerabilities in your marriage from the outset. You need to examine the foundation of this relationship from early on to examine what vulnerabilities may be long-term and how to address them. You also need to adopt a long-term perspective in making sure you give adequate attention to the strengths of this marriage and the reasons for trying to make it work despite the affair. The final exercise for this chapter will help you reflect on the big picture of your relationship as a way of placing the affair in a larger context. But for now, consider the following questions.

Why Did We Become a Couple?

What attracted you and your partner to each other? Most people list a number of factors, from finding the other person easy to talk to and being physically attracted, to sharing fun times together or having a good sexual relationship. They may have discovered common interests, had similar backgrounds, or shared important values. Beyond an initial attraction and subsequent courtship, what led to your decision to marry or commit to one another? Do you value the same parts of the relationship now as you did then? Did you each have good values for selecting a partner, but misjudge how well your partner matched them?

Relationships mature and need to accommodate change, just as people do. You may have entered your relationship based on qualities your partner had that fit the relationship well then but don't serve it as well now. Maybe your relationship took root in your spontaneity and delight in playing together—but now your relationship depends more on your ability to plan and put off play to tend to children or maintain the household. Were there initial sources of attraction or reasons for marrying that weren't entirely healthy? For example, was either of you drawn to the other primarily from feelings of loneliness? Attraction to wealth or status? Fear of growing older without a partner or children? Or you may recognize now that there were early warning signs in your relationship that you either missed or ignored. For example, maybe your courtship was erratic, with repeated breakups or threats to end the relationship.

No partner is perfect. Successful marriages are those in which partners grow together despite their shortcomings, care for each other despite their flaws and differences, and nurture their respective strengths in order to hold on to the good and minimize the bad in their relationship. What were the good qualities that drew you to each other? Were there fundamental flaws in your relationship or in each other that you overlooked?

Can you recover the best parts of your relationship and each other that, at one time, made you want to spend the rest of your lives together?

How Satisfied Were We with Our Respective Roles?

You or your partner may have married with one set of expectations, only to discover later that your experience ended up quite different. The arrival of children, financial setbacks, or unexpected challenges related to physical health or other concerns can all dramatically change partners' roles in and outside their home. Many times partners haven't discussed their respective expectations about such marital and parental roles prior to marrying. Other times the best-laid plans are disrupted by circumstances that neither one of you could have anticipated.

Having your expectations disappointed, and having those disappointments outweigh the satisfactions or fulfillment from your relationship, can easily lead to discontent or resentment. It's sometimes difficult to resolve these conflicts because the choices may be complicated by competing values. Perhaps you both want your young children to be cared for in your home, but you both also believe in the importance of pursuing your own career and supporting your partner's career. Consider the roles you and your partner have most recently had as wage earner, homemaker, spouse, parent, or caretaker for another person. Has either of you felt frustrated or believed you had less opportunity than the other in areas that were important to you? Were you able to talk about these challenges in ways that felt mutually understanding and supportive? If you're particularly unhappy with the roles you've had, what would you need to do to change these roles and what assistance would you need from your partner?

What Have We Done Best?

What stand out as the best parts of your marriage? Despite the trauma of an affair and earlier struggles, couples can often identify parts of their relationship that stand out as particularly worthwhile or special. For some couples, the best part has been the rearing of their children together. For others, it may involve working as a team to build a business or create a comfortable home. For some, the best parts of their marriage have been about friendship or mutual support during times of crisis. What would you have missed out on if you hadn't married each other? What would you miss if you ended your relationship now?

As you reflect on the successes in your marriage, how did these come about? For example, did some of the best qualities seem to come about simply by being yourselves? "Spontaneous" successes often reflect common interests, values, or personality styles that allow collaboration and emotional connection to come about fairly easily. By comparison, past successes that have resulted from conscious effort and determination may be one indicator of how able you are as a couple to work together to overcome the consequences of this affair and address factors that contributed to it.

It will probably require hard work to put this marriage back on solid ground again, if that's the course you decide to pursue. There may be times when you feel as though you're losing ground rather than gaining. However, it may be easier to maintain efforts to rebuild your marriage if you can recall some of your best times in the past as well as how you managed to achieve them.

What Challenges Have We Overcome?

Prior to the affair, you and your partner may already have gone through times that were difficult or challenging. For example, you may have faced financial crises, high demands from rearing young children, dealing with physical illness in a family member, loss of a job, or a move to a different part of the country. For some couples, such challenges strain the relationship in ways that weaken it or leave lasting disappointments or resentments. However, more often couples can look back on such occasions with some satisfaction in recognizing that they withstood the challenge and emerged stronger.

What have been the most difficult times you and your partner have faced together before this affair? What strategies did you draw on as a couple to make it through your most challenging times? Can you recall times in the past when either one of you felt deeply hurt or disappointed by the other? If so, how did you deal with those occasions? You may never before have experienced a hurt in your relationship that comes close to the wound you're suffering now. Nevertheless, thinking about times when you've been able to work through hurt feelings together and to forgive each other in the past—even for lesser relationship injuries—may offer insight into strategies you could draw on as a couple for working through this crisis.

How Does the Current Crisis Fit into the Big Picture?

We've heard both our colleagues and our clients say, "The best predictor of future behavior is past behavior." While there's some truth to this statement, people *are* capable of change. When injured partners struggle to determine whether their marriage could ever feel secure again, we encourage them to look at the big picture of their relationship. Has your partner been faithful and truthful in the past prior to this affair? Has he or she been able to take responsibility for hurtful actions in the past and successfully commit to changing? If relationship problems left your marriage more vulnerable to an affair, are these problems fairly recent or have they been there from the very beginning?

If you're the person who had the affair, you also need to view your marriage and your partner within the bigger picture. The emotional turmoil and conflict that follow an affair may not be an accurate sampling of what your marriage was like before the affair, or what it could be like down the road if you and your partner decide to stay together and work through this challenge. It's not fair to your partner and not in your own best interests to make a decision about what to do with your marriage based on what's going on now. A better basis for evaluating the future requires looking at the big picture of how your marriage has been in the past—including times that felt the best as well as times when you struggled together through the worst.

What Would It Take to Build a Strong Marriage Now?

After long hours of exploring how their marriage had become vulnerable, Kathy and Paul discovered that they had drifted apart while each of them had been trying to care for the marriage in the ways they knew best. Neither one had intended to neglect the other. Kathy recognized that by allowing herself to become totally absorbed in her role at home she had cut herself off from important sources of emotional support from other moms and friends she had known from work. She began to schedule lunches and occasional outings with her friends to balance her need for separate time with Paul with opportunities to receive support from other women. Kathy also learned to approach Paul in a softer tone when con-

veying her needs for closeness, and to provide him encouragement when he felt overwhelmed at work or ineffective at home. Paul worked hard at being more receptive to suggestions from Kathy about how to handle the boys when they were upset or difficult to manage. He also learned to listen more supportively to Kathy's feelings of frustration without becoming defensive or feeling he was necessarily to blame.

Over time, Paul and Kathy began to rebuild their marriage. They restored time for themselves that they had lost to the pressures of work and rearing children. Projects around the house were put off or pursued at a slower pace. They made relationship time a priority. Together they reached decisions regarding finances and child care that allowed Kathy to resume a role in their business one afternoon each week while Paul took the boys on a prearranged outing. At first their discussions about sexual intimacy were quite difficult; Kathy's desire for sex had never been as strong as Paul's, and he found it especially hurtful that she had been sexual with someone else at the same time she was rebuffing his own advances. But with Kathy's encouragement, Paul found better ways of connecting with her emotionally throughout the day—touches in the morning, brief calls in the afternoon, a hug to greet each other in the evening—in ways that increased her desire for lovemaking; at the same time, Kathy looked for opportunities to initiate lovemaking when she felt particularly close to Paul.

During the first six months both Paul and Kathy continued to wrestle with difficult feelings of hurt, guilt, and apprehension about their future together. Their relationship went through numerous ups and downs. But their commitment and efforts at identifying vulnerabilities in their marriage and implementing critical changes eventually paid off. A year after Kathy's affair, they had worked through the crisis and had used the experience as a way of reconstructing their roles in the home and growing closer as a couple.

As you've examined the workings of your relationship, what vulnerabilities have you identified? What relationship strengths have you also recognized—either now or in the past? What would it require from you to reduce or eliminate each source of vulnerability? What would it require from your partner or from the two of you working together? How could you recover or build on strengths in your relationship? Ultimately, your marriage won't work well unless both of you are committed to working on it together. But if you want your marriage to succeed, or if you're not yet sure that you want to end it, for now we encourage you to determine everything you can do on your own to strengthen this relationship regardless of your partner's decisions.

We often tell couples that building a strong marriage requires two kinds of work: reducing hurtful exchanges and initiating positive ones. For now, unless you're already committed to ending your marriage, identify everything you can do on your own to reduce unnecessary conflict and to create an environment that enables both you and your partner to achieve greater fulfillment in your roles both in and outside the home. Then commit yourself to implementing as many changes as you can on your own for a specific time period (for example, 30 or 90 days). During this time, look for opportunities to work on the relationship together with your partner, and use every chance you find to work together. When the opportunities aren't there, try to work on behalf of the relationship on your own. A useful way of communicating your intentions to your partner may be something like this:

> *"I know that this is a really difficult time for us. I still want us to see whether we can find a way of making our marriage work. For now, I'm going to work hard at being a better partner. Sometimes I'll probably fall short, but I'm going to continue trying anyway. I'm also hoping that a part of you still wants our marriage to work, too, and that there will be ways that we can work together. I'll try to be clearer about what I need from you, and I hope you'll be open about what you need from me."*

As you work on strengthening your marriage, look for evidence that your efforts are having an impact. For example, do you feel better about yourself, have greater confidence in your ability to influence what's happening in your life, or respect yourself more? Do your efforts appear to be having an impact on your partner? For example, are there occasions when you experience less anger or more warmth from your partner? Have you acknowledged your partner's efforts as a way of encouraging them further? What impact are your efforts having on your relationship? Are your conflicts any less frequent or less intense? Are there any ways in which you and your partner seem closer or have been more able to work together as a team?

Anticipate that any progress you make in your relationship will be accompanied by occasional setbacks. If you can hang in there and get through these, you and your partner may be able to make some important and lasting positive steps toward building a stronger relationship together.

What's Next?

Work through the following exercises, which follow up on the questions we've posed in this chapter. As indicated in the other chapters, if your partner isn't working with you or willing to examine relationship issues related to the affair at all, remember that your continuing efforts may inspire your partner to join in at some point. Meanwhile, you'll feel better about yourself if you've done everything you can on your own to examine and strengthen the relationship. In Chapter 8, we'll help you to examine what was going on outside your marriage that potentially placed it at greater risk.

———————— Exercises ————————

To make any relationship as good as it can be, you want to keep negative aspects to a minimum while building on what's good. These exercises will help you do that. Some parts of the exercises will help you simply understand your relationship, while other parts will encourage you to do things to improve it. If you already know you're going to stay in your current relationship or think you might, then start making changes now or as soon as you can to improve your relationship. If you're really uncertain about the future of your relationship or it doesn't yet feel safe enough to start working on it, work through the exercises anyway and plan for what you could do in the future if you decide to stay together. You need to develop concrete strategies of how you'll move forward if you do stay together.

EXERCISE 7.1. IDENTIFYING AND DEALING WITH CONFLICT

Even if there are many good things about your relationship, it's hard to enjoy your relationship fully if there also are major conflicts between you.

It's important to identify the areas or issues in your relationship that frequently lead to conflict, and then to develop a plan for addressing those areas more productively.

Identify major sources of conflict in your relationship, whether these are certain aspects of either one of you, how you interact as a couple, or how you interact with people outside your relationship. Clarify which of these conflicts were present prior to the affair and which ones have emerged since then. For example, perhaps you've always struggled with conflict over how to save or spend money or about what to do when one of your parents offers advice on how to rear your children. Or perhaps more recently you've argued about which of you will be responsible for various tasks in your home.

Recognizing what creates conflict between the two of you is important, but doing something about it is critical if you want to stay in your relationship and make it as good as possible. *For each of the sources of conflict you identified earlier, describe what you can do, either individually or as a couple, to address the conflict more effectively.* For example, if a major conflict involves how each partner's mother gets too involved in your child rearing, you might decide that each of you will have an individual talk with your own mother about how you're trying to rear your children and what she can do to support you, along with what's not helpful.

EXERCISE 7.2. PROMOTING EMOTIONAL AND PHYSICAL INTIMACY

Although minimizing conflict is important, one of the true joys of being in a committed relationship comes from feeling intimate with your partner, both emotionally and physically. Partners feel close emotionally from working and playing together, and by sharing their thoughts and feelings with each other—either about what's happening right now or about their dreams for the future.

List the major ways that you and your partner have interacted in the past that led to feeling emotionally close. Some of these may have been disrupted by the affair, but think back to your relationship before that time. For example:

"I often felt closest when we just got silly with each other around the house. Sometimes when music is playing in the background and we're doing routine tasks, we'll break into dance in a very dramatic way, and then we go back to our chores. I could never do that with anyone else."

There might also be ways of feeling close that you haven't developed in the past, or that you'd like to develop further. *List ways you'd like to explore for creating more emotional closeness and specific plans for developing these.* For example:

"When we first got together, we talked about our dreams and what we wanted for a life together. Now, with jobs and kids, we just try to get through the day. If we're going to have any chance of making it, we need to create a new future together. I want us to sit down at least once a month and 'dream' together over a cup of coffee with no one else around."

People in a committed relationship often feel close through their physical relationship.
List the major ways that you and your partner have been physically affectionate in the past that led to feelings of closeness. For example:

"One of my favorite times has been in the mornings when we first wake up. We set the alarm for 15 minutes before we really had to get up, and we snuggled. I need that as a way to start the day and feel connected when we're apart."

Now list the ways that you'd like to strengthen your ways of showing affection. For example:

"We've never tended to show much physical affection, even before the affair. It seems to be sex or nothing. I'd really like it if we just held hands when we're walking someplace. And I've noticed that when we're home and watching television, we sit in separate chairs. I'd like to sit close together on the sofa or lie in bed together and watch our favorite shows."

What do you like or enjoy about your sexual relationship that you want to continue? For example:

"I like it that we don't force lovemaking if either of us is tired, distracted, or not in the mood. I like it that we accept each other's feelings and don't make it into a huge deal."

Now list major areas of concern or areas that need improvement in your sexual relationship and what you can do to improve it. For example:

"I'm glad we're both sensitive to when one of us isn't interested in sex for whatever reason. But more and more, it seems that either one of us is tired, distracted, or needs to work. At least once in a while I'd like to try planning to make love ahead of time, so we can set aside a better time and not be tired or distracted."

EXERCISE 7.3. BUILDING ON STRENGTHS

One of the best ways to improve a relationship is to build on what you do well already. All couples have strengths, and it's important to recognize these and use them in difficult times such as this.

List the major strengths that you have as a couple. This might involve how you've assumed various roles in the relationship, how you parent your children, how you've handled crises in the past, or how each of you supports the other when that person is struggling. For example, you might experience:

"When there's a crisis that's not between us, we generally handle it well. We both figure out what needs to be done, discuss it, and do it in an unselfish way."

Or

"We both understand our responsibilities on a daily basis, and we both follow through very well—either together or individually."

Describe how you can build on these strengths to help you during this difficult time and in the future. For example:

"Since the affair, things have pretty much fallen apart on a day-to-day basis. Things just aren't getting done, which makes everything feel worse. In spite of the bad feelings right now, we need to get back to assuming our regular tasks and responsibilities. We both need some order and predictability right now."

Or

"In the past when things have been tough, we've always turned to our faith to help us get through it. If you can't lean on your faith in tough times, what good is it? We need to go back to church."

8

Was It the World Around Us?

Like many couples, Ira and Hannah struggled to keep up with their busy lives. Full-time jobs and three children left no time for a social life and barely allowed them to go out for dinner or a movie every few weeks. Ira had taken on extra jobs in his remodeling business in anticipation of their oldest son's college expenses starting next year. He rarely made it home for dinner but still tried to make the kids' ball games and recitals. Hannah spent evenings monitoring the kids' homework and catching up on chores after a full day teaching chemistry. The family managed to make Friday night services at the temple most weeks, but Ira and Hannah had dropped out of committees and other congregational activities they valued.

After 19 years of marriage, Ira and Hannah knew they loved each other, and they rarely argued. But they felt like the proverbial ships that pass in the night. Their conversations were generally limited to the business of running the household, and their sex life had all but evaporated. A couple of times recently they had talked about their drifting apart and resolved to change things, but outside demands always seemed to interfere, and they just felt too tired and stressed to dredge up extra energy for a goal that had quickly seemed like just another burden.

Ira's current remodeling job had introduced him to Rebecca, whose husband was often away on business trips. Rebecca showed great appreciation for Ira's craftsmanship, and on his breaks they talked endlessly about the newest home designs and custom furnish-

ings. Over time, they also began to talk about their marriages and their frustrations, although they were clear with each other about being committed to their marriages. Their affair seemed to sneak up on them after weeks of looking through interior design books together, laughing at each other's jokes, sitting a bit too close, and then touching hands a bit longer than necessary when Rebecca passed materials to Ira as she watched him work. When their relationship eventually became sexual, both expressed guilt; at different times both tried to pull back from the affair, but each time they felt drawn back in.

Hannah sensed a growing distance between herself and Ira. He just never seemed emotionally present when he got home. When he started coming home later and later and stopped talking to her once he arrived, Hannah couldn't help feeling nervous. She finally confronted Ira, and he confessed to the affair but insisted he would break it off if only Hannah would forgive him. Neither Ira nor Hannah wanted their marriage to end. They just weren't sure they could ever make it right again.

When people wed and vow to remain faithful to one another for the rest of their lives, they usually mean it. Ira certainly did. So did Rebecca. But marriages become vulnerable. They can become weakened from outside just as they can be weakened from within.

Time can be an insidious force. During the first few years of marriage, and certainly before you're married, your life together is relatively simple. There may not be very many demands on your funds, the prechildren years leave you plenty of time for each other, and possibly your careers haven't imposed a lot of responsibilities and expectations yet. You're probably young and healthy, you may not have made commitments to your community, and your parents are not at the stage of their lives where they're beginning to depend on you.

Enter time and all of the intrusive complications it brings. If you have children now, we don't have to tell you how much time and energy they need and deserve. We don't have to list the expenses that you've added to your budget or the obligations you've added to your daily schedule. Life has become fuller but also possibly harder.

In and of themselves, these normal, predictable challenges are rarely fatal to a marriage. However, when several occur in combination, such stresses and challenges can take a heavy toll on the amount and quality of time that partners have for their own relationship. Exercise 8.1 will help you identify outside negative influences that potentially placed your relationship at higher risk for an affair.

In considering outside factors that can intrude on a relationship, ask yourself the following:

- How did time and energy devoted elsewhere place our marriage at risk?
- How can we take back ownership of our lives to minimize these intrusions in order to safeguard and nurture our marriage?

How Did Outside Intrusions Come between Us?

Work

People vary in how much their work outside the home defines how they feel about themselves. When work forms a large part of your identity or how you see yourself, it's easy for that part of life to dominate other parts. Maybe you spend longer hours at work, or you take work home. Even when you're not actually "working" while at home, how often have you found your mind caught up with what happened at the office or with planning for tomorrow's meeting? Many of us have a hard time leaving the job at the workplace even though we've shut the office door behind us. It's no surprise, then, that our partners sometimes find us distracted or emotionally unavailable.

Work can be seductive. Sometimes we understand better how to do our work than how to be a parent or the kind of husband or wife our partners want us to be. And the rewards from work are sometimes more immediate and more tangible. If we're productive, we get a good evaluation and perhaps a raise. We're encouraged to work hard and get ahead. The harder we work and the more we achieve, often the more responsibility we're given and the more time and energy are required to meet those responsibilities. It can easily become a vicious cycle. The harder we work and the more successful we are, the greater the incentives to work harder still to achieve even more success—whether this means achieving financial rewards, recognition from others, or simply a sense of personal accomplishment.

In our work as couple therapists, our clients often tell us they work so hard because they have to. They have to support the family. They're in a cutthroat work environment, and only the people working 60 to 70 hours a week still have a job. If they let up, they and their families will suffer. The bills won't get paid. There will be fewer family vacations. College for their children will be out of the question, or they'll have to attend second-rate schools. In most cases there's just enough truth in each of these assertions to create a sense of being trapped. After all, bills *do* have to get paid, and in some settings you either get promoted or you get fired. But in every case there's also a choice being made. If moving to a smaller home and reducing your mortgage payments meant you could spend more time with your partner in nurturing your marriage, would it be worth it? If by working so hard to support your family you end up *losing* your family because your marriage becomes more vulnerable to an affair, is that worth it?

Knowing that, as with many things in life, you can't have it all, what are you willing to give up in terms of your work for the sake of your marriage? If worse came to worst, how willing would you be to risk your job to preserve your marriage? Short of that, what limits are you willing to set on the time and energy you devote to work in order to redirect your focus to nurturing your relationship? What specific steps would you have to take to implement these limits? How can you increase support at work or at home for your decision to place your marriage as your highest priority?

Responsibilities of Rearing Children

Next to work, rearing children is the most frequently cited demand on couples' time. And each stage of child rearing intrudes on relationship time in different ways. As therapists, we emphasize to couples that rearing children can be so demanding and so exhausting that the *only* way to do this well is to make sure that the couple preserves time and energy for their own marriage. *The best gift that parents can give to their children is a secure home in which the parents love and nurture one another as an example of a loving relationship for their children. Placing your marriage at risk by devoting all your time and energy to your children at the expense of partners' caring for each other just doesn't make good sense.* Parents need to risk their children's frustrations or disappointments in the short run by setting aside time for themselves as a couple in order to strengthen their marriage and promote their children's well-being in the long run.

Balancing your commitments to your children and to your marriage requires continuous effort. It may require partnering with other couples to trade evenings of providing child care. It often requires helping your children respect their parents' privacy and need for separate time apart before joining in family time. Above all, it requires a steady commitment to setting aside quality time for you and your partner and placing your marriage as a top priority—not because you don't care about your children, but specifically because you *do* care for them and recognize that the strength of your marriage is one of the most important assets your children have.

In what ways have the demands of child rearing disrupted time and energy you and your partner set aside for your marriage? If you've allowed your children to participate in so many activities outside of school that these consume your available time as well as theirs, how can you scale back? What resources can you draw on to provide respite and opportunities to focus on your marriage? For example, are there couples you know from work, school, or your neighborhood with whom you could occasionally trade evenings of watching the children? What steps could you take to ensure that you and your partner have at least 15 minutes of quiet time together each day to talk by yourselves and reconnect with each other?

Outside Commitments

It's not just work or children that compete for your time and energy, obviously. Numerous organizations depend on the contributions of volunteers: your children's schools, your religious group, and various community service organizations. Just like paid positions, volunteer work can contribute a lot to our sense of self-worth. At appropriate levels, the satisfaction derived from contributing to such causes can not only enrich individual lives but can also bring outside energy into the home and marriage. As with work, however, it's a matter of balance and priorities.

How much time do you and your partner devote to commitments outside the home other than work? In what ways have such commitments interfered with time for your marriage? What commitments would you be willing to give up for the sake of your relationship? What limits would you need to set on remaining commitments to reduce the risks posed to your marriage by spending too much time apart?

Responsibilities to Extended Family

For many couples, partners' respective families of origin provide an important source of emotional and other support. For other couples, involvement with extended family sometimes places additional demands or strains on a marriage. It's not uncommon for partners to have different expectations about how much time or energy either one should devote to his or her own or to the other's extended family. Such differences can lead to resentment about feeling less of a priority in the other's life, or about feeling denied the opportunity to hold on to important emotional ties with one's family.

Another way in which responsibilities to extended family can strain a couple's relationship occurs when one or the other partner takes on a caregiving role for someone in the extended family. A common example involves caring for an aging parent, but it can just as easily involve caring for grandparents or for siblings with physical or mental disabilities. As therapists, we have found that most of the couples we've worked with, in which one or both partners also care for someone in the extended family, have a profound sense of responsibility deeply rooted in admirable family values. However, as in caring for their children, it's important to maintain a balance that also protects and nurtures the couple's own relationship.

In what ways have your or your partner's involvement with extended family detracted from the time and energy you've devoted to your own relationship? How much of this involvement came in response to expectations rather than need—for example, times when extended family wanted you to be with them when it might have been more important to preserve that time for yourselves? If your involvement with extended family comes from caregiving responsibilities, how can you redesign your roles to set reasonable limits that will preserve vital emotional and time resources for your marriage? If you want to care for extended family as well as your marriage, what additional resources can you draw on to balance these commitments more effectively?

Household Tasks

All couples have ongoing responsibilities in the home as well as outside. Obvious tasks include laundry, cleaning, meals, house or car maintenance, yard work, paying the bills, and so forth. Managing these tasks while dealing with competing responsibilities of child rearing or work outside the home can be difficult. Even when you two agree on how to divide or share these responsibilities, getting everything done while preserving quality time for your marriage can seem impossible. When you disagree on how to share these tasks or one feels the other isn't upholding his or her end of the bargain, resentment often follows.

You and your partner might agree on how to divide household tasks but disagree on how to get them done and how important doing so is as compared with reserving time simply to relax or play together. Your standard for housecleaning may require an entire day each weekend, whereas your partner is content with what can be accomplished in an hour or two. One of you may be comfortable making love with dirty laundry scattered about in the bedroom and dishes in the sink, whereas the other can't enjoy lovemaking while there are still chores to be done.

In thinking about how you and your partner manage household tasks, consider these questions: Do you generally agree on how to divide up household tasks, or does either of you frequently feel you do more than your share? How willing are you to put work at home aside in order to preserve time to relax and play together? What tasks could you give up? Which ones could you hire out? How could you and your partner collaborate to balance work and play at home in ways that feel better for both of you?

Hobbies and Similar Interests

Hobbies and leisure activities can reduce stress and increase emotional and physical well-being, make a person more interesting to be around, and even provide common ground for shared leisure when the two of you are interested in the same thing. But they can become a distraction when they take up too much time, especially when you already have too little time for each other.

Toni loved the energy and attractive figure she achieved by exercising, so she devoted an hour after work to it and at least half a day each weekend. Alex resented the time he spent alone at home but didn't want to join Toni because he didn't like working out and was intimidated by the other guys at the gym who seemed to be in much better shape. Alex had always had an interest in rebuilding cars, and at first he pursued this interest by reconditioning a friend's van in their garage. Then he started spending more time with other guys who liked working on old cars, and soon he and his friends were traveling on weekends to auto shows out of town. Neither Alex nor Toni wanted to give up their own outside interests, even when it became clear they were spending too little time together for several weeks in a row.

In what ways have you or your partner allowed hobbies or similar interests to come between you, and how could you change that? Could you schedule them for times you and your partner are already likely to be apart? How willing are you to scale back the amount of time you devote to separate interests? Could either of you become more accepting of separate hobbies if you were also spending more time together? Are there ways of pursuing your separate interests at the same time or in the same space?

How Did Stress Overcome Us?

Low levels of stress and more acute but temporary stressors are often manageable and can even be positive if such a stressor causes you to think or behave in new ways that are better for you in the long run. But when stress is severe or long-term, it can cause bigger and longer-lasting problems, including in your relationship.

Excessive or prolonged stress can place a marriage at higher risk for an affair when the stressors cause partners to neglect themselves or their marriage. Sometimes a partner under duress tries to escape emotionally into the comfort of an affair relationship that is largely sheltered from day-to-day realities. Other times a partner overwhelmed by stress becomes emotionally or physically unavailable so that the other feels abandoned and ends up vulnerable to the attentions of someone else. When stress permeates a household, both partners can become irritable and impatient, desperate to fault each other for problems neither is really responsible for, and gradually they decline into a cycle of mutual blame and resentment.

Common sources of stress that can undermine a relationship include:

- Chronic financial strains.
- Difficult life transitions—for example, becoming parents or starting a new job.
- Chronic health problems.
- Ongoing conflicts with others—for example, with extended family or co-workers.

Over the past year, how did excessive stress make your marriage vulnerable? Which stressors developed gradually or escaped your notice until it seemed too late? What would be required now to reduce or eliminate the sources of greatest stress? What additional resources can you draw on for help?

> *Ira and Hannah, the couple described at the beginning of this chapter, took a hard look at how they had allowed external demands and stressors to erode the emotional foundation of their marriage. In trying so hard to be responsible providers for their family, they had neglected to care for their marriage. Both Ira and Hannah acknowledged that they had each contributed to the marriage's vulnerability to outside influences. In response, each worked to impose more effective limits on their work; Hannah gave up supervising an after-school science club, and Ira no longer accepted remodeling jobs that took him away from the family at night. Costs of college didn't seem quite as daunting after meeting with a financial aid officer at their community college; replacing Ira's aging truck could be put off another year or two after a mechanic agreed to work on it in exchange for Ira's building a new workbench and cabinets in his garage. They also reassigned responsibilities in the home to each of the children—including having their oldest son babysit for his younger siblings one night each week so his parents could go out by themselves. Ira and Hannah identified certain days during the week that were particularly stressful for one of them or the other, and agreed to exchange "care days" on those occasions so each could get some relief when he or she needed it most. They also pursued more touching and hugging throughout the day, recognizing that such closeness promoted stronger desire in each of them for more frequent sexual intimacy. Their increased commitment to nurturing their marriage didn't by itself solve the deep hurt caused by Ira's affair, but it gave both partners increased hope that they could collaborate in creating a stronger relationship and moving forward together.*

Did We Let Others Undermine Our Marriage?

Although wedding vows differ across societies and religions, nearly all include promises of fidelity—"forsaking all others"—regardless of the circumstances (as in "for richer or poorer, in sickness or in health"). It's ironic, then, how frequently sexual infidelity is portrayed in our culture as commonplace, romantic, rejuvenating, justifiable, and often without negative effects. At times infidelity almost seems taken for granted—depicted in a glamorous or even comical way—rather than being portrayed in a more realistic manner as a relationship trauma with devastating personal and relationship consequences. Anyone's commitment to marital fidelity can be undermined when continually exposed to this perspective.

Jay was one of the few men at his firm who was married. Most of the men his own age were still single; some of the older men were divorced. On Fridays after work they all had a ritual of going out to dinner together at a local club. Often the other guys would flirt shamelessly with women at the club and would tease Jay about being "tied down" by marriage and missing out on life. At first Jay laughed at their jokes, but privately he was glad he was married. He loved his wife, Cindy, and couldn't imagine a life without her. But things started to change after Cindy got pregnant and the baby arrived. She complained about the time Jay spent with his friends, even though when he was home she seemed to ignore him and spend all her time with the baby. Money was a big problem, now that Cindy had quit her job. The baby struggled with colic and never seemed comforted when Jay held her. His friends at work teased him even more when he talked about the problems at home. One of his friends and two women from work invited him out for drinks one evening, and eventually they were going out once a week. Jay suspected that his friend and one of the women were sexually involved, although they never said so directly. The other woman—Alice—recently divorced, paid lots of attention to Jay and made him feel desirable in ways that he no longer felt with Cindy.

One evening Jay and Alice went out after work for drinks by themselves when their friends weren't available. Jay didn't intend for anything to happen between him and Alice—he just enjoyed talking with her. She made him laugh and she always commented on how well he was doing in the office. Eventually he and Alice were going out after work every few weeks by themselves. When Alice invited Jay over to her apartment instead of going to the club, he felt flattered. He knew that Alice found him attractive—she had practically come right out and told him so. When they got to her apartment and she kissed him, he was a bit surprised by her taking the initiative but wasn't offended. The kiss felt good. But then she wanted more. At first Jay resisted; he knew it was wrong. But he and Cindy hadn't been intimate since early in her pregnancy. Alice insisted she wasn't looking for any kind of commitment and said she didn't want to hurt Jay's marriage. But she continued to hold him, caress his neck, and eventually led him to her bedroom. That was the first of several such instances that continued for several months.

People like Jay, with no intention of becoming involved in an affair, often become more vulnerable after repeated exposure to innuendo, suggestion, or outright pursuit by an outsider. Unfortunately, they often don't notice this happening. Only with 20-20 hindsight do they see, once they've had an affair, all the temptations and fidelity-undermining messages they've been barraged with. It's worth examining the common sources of temptations and other negative influences discussed below to see which contributed to the affair that disrupted your marriage so that you or your partner won't be so vulnerable to these forces again. As the injured partner, you'll benefit from understanding the risk factors that contributed to your partner's affair and should certainly read this section. But most of it is aimed at encouraging participating partners to explore how they may have failed to set boundaries that would prevent outside influences from undermining their commitment to fidelity. When we say "you" here, we're speaking to participating partners.

General Temptations and Opportunity

In working with participating partners, we sometimes ask, "How did you reach your decision to have an affair?" A common response is, "I never decided to have an affair—it just happened." Our next question—admittedly more difficult to answer—is then, *"Well, how is it you failed to reach a decision not to have an affair?"* The implication is that you can identify risky situations ahead of time and take explicit steps to avoid these. Consider the following situations that present either temptation or opportunity for an affair:

- Frank's work in sales frequently requires him to travel to cities in which he has no friends, family, or colleagues. After working long days, he usually has dinner at a local bar or dance club.
- Sally has been spending lots of time over the past few months preparing for a school carnival with Gerald, a single parent whose work schedule allows him to spend much of his day at home.

- Tuan and Linh have been working nights and weekends at the office preparing for a major trade convention. No one else is involved in the project, and sometimes they take time out at the restaurant down the street before returning to work—without informing their spouses later.

Do any of these situations have elements that seem familiar? We're not suggesting that any of these scenarios is inherently wrong, but we *are* saying that people need to recognize the possible temptations in a situation—no matter how far-fetched they may seem ahead of time—and then set clear boundaries to ensure that temptations don't lead to poor decisions. For example, if you're traveling alone, do you make it a point to call your partner regularly to stay emotionally connected and to keep your relationship at the forefront of your thoughts? If your partner is frequently out of town, do you draw on same-sex friends in committed marriages to keep you company or to socialize? If your work or involvement in the community results in your spending time with a coworker of the opposite sex, have you taken steps to ensure that feelings of personal closeness don't develop to an inappropriate level or cascade into feelings of strong sexual attraction? For example, do you limit—rather than tolerate or promote—opportunities for highly personal discussions or other intimate exchanges with your coworker that lead to an inappropriate level of intimacy?

Take a hard, close look at how you and your partner spend your time whenever you're apart. What opportunities might either of you face that could increase the risk of infidelity? Remember that identifying such situations doesn't indicate your interest in an affair; rather, identifying potentially risky situations and taking active measures to minimize and guard against them conveys your commitment *not* to have an affair and to remove any possible opportunity or temptation to behave in ways that are contrary to your interests and values.

Pursuit by an Outsider

It feels good to feel attractive or desirable. We all like to receive compliments. "Innocent" flirtation often feels good for similar reasons. It's often reassuring to know that someone else considers us bright, charming, witty, successful, emotionally sensitive, caring, strong, physically attractive, supportive, or whatever other characteristic we'd like to believe about ourselves. It feels especially good to receive such compliments when we tend to have self-doubts or haven't been receiving such comments from our partner.

It's not unusual to be drawn into an affair following pursuit by someone outside the relationship. Such pursuit may develop gradually over months or even years of interaction, or it may come quite unexpectedly from an acquaintance. The pursuit may begin with an explicit intention by the other to have an affair or as a genuine wish to have a special friendship based on caring and trust that subsequently leads to feelings of physical attraction. Sometimes an outsider persists despite clear, explicit resistance and discouragement. And other times a pursuit continues because of an individual's tolerance or subtle encouragement.

If you're uncertain whether an outside relationship has begun to edge toward a "special" friendship that poses a risk, ask yourself the following:

- Would you be willing to give up this outside friendship for the sake of your marriage? If not, there's a good chance that it has already developed a "specialness" that threatens emotional or physical bonds that your partner expects to be unique to your own relationship.
- Would you be willing to confront the other person about the "mixed signals" you're getting about the boundaries of your friendship—knowing that he or she might very well pull back from the relationship you're currently enjoying? Are there elements of flirtation or emotional closeness that have already become something you look forward to and would miss if they ended?
- Are there *any* aspects of your interactions with the outside person you'd be reluctant for your partner to know about? Are there any discussions you would not disclose fully to your partner? Are there any times when interacting with the outside person that you'd be uncomfortable in receiving a phone call from your partner?

To reduce vulnerability to outsiders who may wish to pursue an affair—or who may simply be "receptive" to such a relationship—it's important to maintain appropriate vigilance. That doesn't mean rejecting all friendships with colleagues and others. It doesn't mean rejecting all expressions of caring or interpreting them as implicit sexual advances. But it does mean being clear about the boundaries of such relationships—that you don't pursue or accept suggestions of separate time together in inappropriate settings, that you guard against personal discussions that push a friendship to a level you can't handle, and that you commit to never keeping interactions with others secret from your partner.

We've counseled people who insisted on their right to retain an outside relationship because it was an "innocent" friendship and was not sexual in nature. In most cases, their very reluctance to relinquish the outside friendship indicated the extent to which the other person had become emotionally important to them and made clear why their partners perceived this "friendship" as a threat to their own relationship. If your partner insists that you have *no* interactions with anyone of the opposite sex outside his presence, there may be problems of trust or jealousy in your own relationship that require some further attention. But if that's not what your partner is demanding, and instead he's raising concerns about a particular outside relationship, there's a possibility that something about that relationship poses a potential risk. This doesn't mean you've decided to have an affair. It's simply that an affair sometimes develops when a person views an outside relationship as "safe" and then gradually becomes more involved with the other person without maintaining necessary limits or boundaries. That relationship then becomes "risky."

Friends and Acquaintances Who Devalue Fidelity

No one has a greater investment in preserving your marriage than you and your partner do. Unfortunately, not only may your friends or acquaintances fail to actively promote your remaining faithful in your marriage, they may either actively or indirectly discourage it. For example, they may encourage you to stay out or party with them and tease you if you state that you "need to call home" first. They may encourage you to go to singles bars because "a little looking never hurt anyone." They may persuade you to have "a night out on the town" when you are traveling together. Or they may serve as a "go-between" for someone outside your relationship who has expressed an interest in you.

Other means of undermining your fidelity are less direct. For example, your single or divorced friends may talk up all the benefits of being single while ignoring the downside. They may listen to your own stories of marital unhappiness and encourage your disgruntlement or feelings of unfairness by siding with you in an unbalanced way, fanning the flames of your discontent by emphasizing only the negative and none of the positive features of your partner. They may undermine your relationship by competing for time you would otherwise spend with your partner.

Misery Loves Company

Some wrongdoers seek out co-conspirators, and the unhappy can undermine the contented by focusing on the negatives in committed relationships. Be skeptical when such individuals tell you how happy they are that they've escaped the shackles of marriage. Choose your friends and acquaintances carefully. Remember that the short-term gratification that these unhappy individuals claim to get rarely offsets the risks of losing a lifelong partner.

How Should We Draw on Others to Support Our Marriage?

It's not enough to protect yourself from outside influences that increase your relationship's vulnerability to an affair. You also need to seek out support for your marriage from sources that nurture it and *reduce* its vulnerability. What bases of support for fidelity and for your marriage in general are available to you and your partner? Although such assets vary in couples' lives, some common resources are described here. Exercise 8.2 will help you consider specific resources in your own life.

Couple Friends

Developing friendships with other committed couples can provide an important source of caring and support for your own relationship. What couples do you know who enjoy spending time with each other—partners who are courteous to one another, laugh with each other, express their complaints respectfully, tolerate each other's shortcomings, and work together at overcoming occasional disappointments or irritations? Your own relationship can be strengthened by spending time with couples whose values are similar to those you aspire to yourself. Avoid couples who constantly bicker, put each other down, seek laughs at the other's expense, are generally insensitive to one another, or appear to pursue individual interests that put their relationship at risk.

Couple-Oriented Groups

You and your partner can also find support for your relationship by participating in various groups or organizations that encourage committed relationships. Many couples experience such support through active participation in their church or synagogue—particularly through activities that promote small-group interaction where couples can work and play together. Other couples find support in various social organizations that are oriented specifically to couple- or family-based activities—for example, working in the community food bank together on Saturday mornings or going on weekend camping excursions together.

What's Next?

Use the exercises in this chapter not only to reduce outside negative influences, but also to draw on resources around you to support your relationship and your commitment to fidelity. After you've worked through these exercises and have taken specific actions regarding outside influences you've identified as important to your marriage, go on to Chapter 9. The next two chapters build on work you've already done by helping you and your partner look more closely at the two of you as individuals.

———————————— Exercises ————————————

EXERCISE 8.1. IDENTIFYING OUTSIDE NEGATIVE INFLUENCES

Work outside the home, time spent with your children, service to others, and time for yourself are all worthwhile but, when taken to excess or in combination, can interfere with your relationship. In addition to these normal aspects of life, various stresses such as financial burdens, health concerns, and conflict with others can interfere with your relationship. And other people who don't help to support your marriage, such as friends with different values or the outside person who was pursuing one of you, can make your relationship vulnerable to an affair.

List the major factors outside your relationship—intrusions such as work, major stresses such as financial burdens, or other people—that have undermined your relationship. For example, you might have taken on so much in the community with civic or charitable work that you don't have time for your relationship. Or you might realize:

"I really never did think that 'guys' night out' was a good idea with those particular people. They don't share our values about commitment, and they were a bad influence."

Recognizing outside forces that have undermined your relationship is important, but doing something about these is critical if you want to stay in your relationship and make it as good as possible. *For each of the outside factors you listed above that take away from your relationship, describe what you can do, either individually or as a couple, to minimize their effect on your relationship.* For example, you might decide:

"We both value giving back to the community and have always done that, but we've clearly overdone it and left no time and energy for us. I think each of us should limit our outside meetings to no more than one night a week."

EXERCISE 8.2. BUILDING ON OUTSIDE RESOURCES

Just as there were probably factors and people outside your relationship that made it more vulnerable to an affair, there likely are outside factors and people who can help to strengthen your relationship—couple friends, individual friends, and groups that will support your relationship.

List the major people and groups that you can turn to now or have turned to in the past to support and strengthen your relationship. For example:

"My brother-in-law is someone I truly admire. I'd really like to spend more time with him, not to talk about the affair, but just to be with someone whom I can learn from and see how he handles various stresses and how he prioritizes his family. As busy as he is, if he can do it, I can learn to do it, too."

There likely also are people or groups that you haven't taken full advantage of that would support your relationship or help to strengthen it. *List the major people whom you would like to spend more time with and groups you would like to be part of that would support and strengthen your relationship.* For example:

"We're really fortunate to live in a family neighborhood with many couples our age. They have lots of informal get-togethers, but we haven't participated very much. I want to start saying yes to those invitations and have some of the families in the neighborhood over to our house."

How Could My Partner Have Done This?

Nick owned his own company, had paid off his home and two late-model cars, and—at age 43—was aware that women found him physically attractive. He felt confident and had a smile and easy manner that others found both comfortable and engaging.

It hadn't always been that way. Always somewhat small for his age and slow to develop physically, he had been shy and awkward as a teenager. He had hardly dated in high school, and he still remembered somewhat painfully having been turned down for prom in his senior year by three different girls before deciding to stay home. When he finished high school and went to work for his father at the family hardware store while most of his friends moved away to attend college, he had felt stupid and inept.

But he worked hard at his family's business and his father compensated him well. It wasn't long before Nick had more money to play with than most of his friends still in school, and he found it surprisingly easy to impress some of the high school girls with his sense of direction and responsibility. His father helped him start his own electrical contracting business as a part-time venture, and gradually Nick built his own company with about a dozen employees. As the years went by, his naturally trim build helped him stay in shape more easily than lots of men his age. The shyness he had experienced as an ado-

lescent had now grown into a confident but quiet and sensitive manner that women seemed to find attractive.

Nick had married Becky within a month after she graduated from high school and he had turned 21. She was attractive if not gorgeous, and she shared Nick's conservative values and commitment to hard work. Before their first child arrived she worked as a bank teller, and they had established a firm financial footing for their marriage even before Nick's contracting firm took off. Nick admired his wife for all she did for their marriage and their children.

Nick had no interest in chasing other women, but he was flattered that some of them seemed interested in chasing him—despite his making clear that he was married with three children. He never took the flirtation seriously—until Diana came along. She was divorced and owned her own real estate business, and Nick found her a bit intimidating though incredibly attractive. So when she invited him to lunch to discuss renovations to some rental properties she had bought, he felt both flattered and apprehensive. But Diana was reassuring, had a delightful laugh, and complimented Nick on all he had accomplished. She was also openly admiring of how well he had kept himself in shape, and shared with him how easy she found him to talk with. Nick was a bit incredulous when it became clear that she was attracted to him. He had never been unfaithful to Becky and had no intention of doing anything to threaten their marriage. But when Diana made it clear she wasn't looking for a serious relationship with Nick but only wanted some physical intimacy with a man she admired and trusted, he found his feelings overwhelming reason. For six months he and Diana met discreetly at one of her duplexes and had passionate sex, usually followed by an hour or more of snuggling and discussing work. Talk about their personal lives remained generally off-limits.

Just as affairs can happen in a good marriage, affairs can "happen" to good people. Good, loving, and previously faithful partners can make bad decisions that lead them astray. When you decided to marry your partner, it's unlikely that you imagined you would ever experience this kind of betrayal. You trusted your partner not to hurt you in this way. No matter what disagreements you had, no matter what struggles you experienced, you didn't expect to suffer your partner's affair. Now you need to make sense of how the person you loved and trusted could have done this.

In this chapter we're mostly going to help the injured partner consider aspects of the other partner that may have contributed to the affair. If you're the participating partner, we encourage you to read through this chapter, too, to gain insight into your partner's perspective as well as a better understanding of yourself and how you came to have an affair. At the very least, please read "A Special Message to the Participating Partner" on page 208.

How did your partner get involved? If the affair continued beyond one or two occasions, why did your partner persist? If the affair is still going on, why won't your partner just end it? How you answer these questions will be significant to how you decide to move on and how well you're able to carry out whatever relationship decisions you make down the road.

It's important to achieve a *balanced* view of your partner—one that's neither unduly negative and all-condemning nor unrealistically positive and excusing. It's unlikely that the person you fell in love with and chose to marry has no positive qualities, despite having hurt you deeply. "Demonizing" your partner can have several negative consequences. First, if you haven't already completely and irreversibly decided to end your marriage, then you need to consider how you could work to regain a caring and trusting relationship with this person who betrayed you. You won't be able to do this without considering your partner's vulnerabilities that led to an affair with at least some understanding or compassion; you may even need to consider how your partner's affair came about partly because of some of your partner's positive qualities or strengths.

Second, if you want your partner to join you in exploring the context that led to the affair, you're going to have to challenge and perhaps soften your own perspective to make it safe enough for your partner to engage in this process. You may believe that your partner doesn't deserve any consideration or kindness right now. But if what *you* need is to have your partner participate in trying to figure out how this affair came about, you may have to do what's necessary to get this.

A third reason comes into play if you do decide to move on by ending your marriage and if there are children involved. In that case it will be important to continue to collaborate as parents. The research on children's well-being following divorce is very clear on one thing: *The most important factor in children's adjustment to divorce is how effectively their parents can work together after the end of their marriage.* You and your partner will both find it hard to parent together if either one of you views the other as having no positive or redeeming qualities. Finally, if you end your marriage, it will be important for you to make sense of your original decision to marry this person. If you conclude that your partner is purely evil and without any virtues whatsoever, it will be more difficult for you to trust your judgment in future relationship decisions.

A balanced view is important to avoiding the opposite extreme too. Being unduly positive and rushing to "excuse" your partner of responsibility for the affair may feel safer or more comfortable in the short term, because it allows you to regain a sense of closeness or intimacy. But if you don't confront issues regarding your partner now, you're more likely to have lingering doubts that could surface at unexpected moments weeks, months, or even years down the road. By then it will be much more difficult to engage in the exploration process we're encouraging you to pursue now.

As you read through this chapter, consider not only vulnerabilities but also potential strengths or positive aspects of your partner that may have contributed to the affair. Think about how it came about, how or why it continued, and how it ended or has failed to end. Not everything we invite you to consider here will be relevant to your situation. Don't rush to conclusions that may turn out to be inaccurate or incomplete; moreover, pursuing a "personality analysis" of your partner that blames his or her core character for the affair is likely to block any inclination your partner may have to join you in this process. Take your time, consider what you read as possible "hypotheses" for what has happened, and be sure to fit whatever seems to make sense into the larger overall picture that extends beyond your partner to include contributions from your marriage, the outside world, and perhaps even aspects of yourself.

A Special Message to the Participating Partner

If you're working through this book with your injured partner, we commend your decision to participate in this healing process. As we stated in the first chapter, not all participating partners are willing to engage in the difficult and sometimes painful process of examining how the affair came about in order to work toward recovery. If for no other reason, we encourage you to stick with this process because it's what your partner needs from you. Examining the aspects of yourself that made you vulnerable to having an affair may be particularly difficult. It may be hard not to become defensive or to respond with, "Yes, but . . . ": "Yes, but what about the way our marriage was?" "Yes, but what about everything else that was going on?" "Yes, but what about you?" As well as you can for now, try to trust in the overall process that will work toward understanding the big picture. That may help you in taking a hard look at that part of the big picture that involves you. Your partner needs you to do this.

This chapter is also intended to help you sort through your own feelings. In our clinical work, we find that men or women who have participated in an affair often struggle to make sense of their own behavior. "This just isn't like me; how could I have done this?" In struggling to come to grips with their feelings of confusion, guilt, or shame, participating partners sometimes overlook or resist examining parts of themselves that could help them understand how an affair developed. The risk in not doing this is that the explanations they settle on often are incomplete or inaccurate. We've had participating partners conclude, incorrectly, that for them to have done something so hurtful to their injured partners, they must not have really loved them as deeply as they thought. Other times they've decided that the only way to restore dignity to their lives or achieve redemption is to give up the marriage and lead a life of aloneness. Sometimes, by ignoring their own contributions, they've placed too much weight on difficulties in the marriage or on positive qualities of the outside affair person as a reason for the affair and then have made poor long-term relationship choices as a consequence. We want to help you avoid those risks.

We also want you to assess any aspects of yourself that contributed to the affair so that you can reduce any risks of another affair in the future. In all likelihood, you've already promised your partner and yourself never to have another affair, so further examination of how the affair came about doesn't feel necessary. But it's also likely that you never planned on having an affair the first time you pledged to be faithful "for better or worse." We don't question your intentions to remain faithful. But we do have concerns about your ability to carry out your intentions if you avoid looking at important aspects of yourself that potentially placed you at risk.

Finally, if you're still involved in your affair or sometimes have difficulty dealing with its being over, you need to understand everything you can about why these feelings are continuing. Some of what's happening may involve your conflicting needs and feelings that are particularly confusing or difficult to resolve. Reading through this chapter to understand yourself better may help you reach decisions more clearly that are best for you in the long run.

How Could My Partner Have Gotten Involved?

Before you, the injured partner, try to answer this question, we first want to provide you with a way of thinking about factors that might have contributed to your partner's vulnerability to an affair. Some of these may extend well back in time and involve attitudes, beliefs, anxieties, needs, or other tendencies that were in place before you and your partner ever met. Examples might include unrealistic beliefs about how a marriage is supposed to be, lack of confidence in oneself as an intimate partner, or an inability to withstand long periods of unhappiness or stress without much support or relief. Think of such factors as paving the way for an affair. They don't cause an affair to happen, but they can raise the vulnerability or risk of an affair if certain other conditions come along.

Other factors that made the affair more likely to occur may have predated it by only weeks or months, such as flirting with someone who was also susceptible to an affair, developing an emotionally intimate relationship and spending increasing time alone with someone else, or seeking the company of the opposite sex when traveling out of town on business. Such behaviors don't inevitably lead to an affair, but they clearly lower the safeguards and raise the risks.

Finally, there may be factors that "triggered" the affair either separately or in combination with other conditions—from alcohol or other substance use that lowers inhibitions and clouds judgment, to anger toward a partner that leads to an affair as retaliation, or recent loss or trauma that increases the need for comfort or reassurance.

In most cases, answering the question "How could my partner have gotten involved?" requires thinking of all of these kinds of factors—some long-term, others more recent, and some brief or even coincidental. Understanding your partner's vulnerability to an affair involves adopting the larger view. You need to consider not only who your partner *is*, but also how your partner came to be this way and is *likely to be* in the future. Exercise 9.1 will help you consider these factors further.

What Was My Partner Looking For?

Popular myths regarding infidelity suggest that men have affairs to pursue better or more frequent sex and to experience the thrill of seduction and conquest, whereas women have affairs to pursue emotional connection and overcome fears of growing older and becoming less attractive. Like many stereotypes, these beliefs sometimes contain an element of truth but fail to capture a far more complex reality. The reasons for affairs are as varied as the individuals having them, as discussed in the following paragraphs.

Affirmation of Self-Worth

All of us feel neglected or unappreciated at one time or another. But several factors can intensify or perpetuate such feelings in a way that prompts a person to seek the kinds of affirmation sometimes provided by an affair. One is long-standing self-doubt. Like Nick, the husband we described at the opening of this chapter, some people lack confidence in their attractiveness, social status or prestige, importance to others, or more general meaning and purpose in life, and that lack of confidence goes back to adolescence or even earlier. Unresolved self-doubts, a low tolerance for criticism, and high needs for approval and appreciation can sometimes outstrip the capacity of any spouse or marriage to provide nurturing and acceptance as frequently as desired. When this happens, the problem isn't the marriage; rather, the participating partner needs to examine those needs for affirmation and how much they might place unrealistic demands on any marriage.

Comparatively high needs for affirmation can be exacerbated when a couple has reduced opportunities for providing caring and support to one another, such as when both partners work outside the home, a new baby arrives, or one or more children have special needs that place additional demands on their parents. Your partner's need for affirmation can also soar when some event undermines or shakes his feelings of confidence or connectedness: The death of a parent, coworker, or close friend might remind your partner of his mortality and trigger the pursuit of comfort or connection in an affair; so can difficulties at work or the loss of a job, financial setbacks, physical health problems, or an unwanted change in physical appearance.

Was your partner vulnerable to needs for reassurance from someone else? If so, has he always had high needs for such affirmation? Were there situations leading up to the affair that intensified these needs or interfered with their being met within the marriage?

Affirmation of Sexual Attractiveness and Adequacy

Most of us want to feel sexy, desirable, and adequate as sexual partners. When stresses or external demands in the marriage interfere with love-making, or when the sexual relationship suffers from specific problems of its own, anyone can become more vulnerable to seeking sexual fulfillment or affirmation through an affair.

Sometimes people also pursue an affair as a way of exploring aspects of their sexuality that they're uncomfortable pursuing in their marriage. For example, in some cases a man may become particularly aroused by sexual behaviors that he's comfortable pursuing only with someone with whom he's not also emotionally connected, either because he's never revealed this interest to his spouse and hesitates to introduce it so far into their marriage or because he feels anxious or repulsed by the thought that his wife and mother of their children would engage in (or perhaps even enjoy) these "illicit" acts. Similarly, a woman may be apprehensive about taking a more assertive, creative, or passionate sexual role in her marriage if she anticipates that her husband could view this as a threatening change or if she simply feels reticent about introducing a new aspect of herself. It's not unusual for a spouse to feel obligated to behave as he or she always has, because that's the person his or her wife or husband married and anything else may not be considered attractive or even acceptable.

What can you learn from your history together? Has your partner struggled with concerns about her sexual desirability in the past? Have difficulties in your sexual relationship or stresses on the marriage hampered your lovemaking? Has your partner expressed dissatisfaction with your sexual relationship in the past, or have discussions about this aspect of your marriage felt awkward or difficult?

Emotional Connection and Intimacy

Sometimes it's the pursuit of emotional intimacy that sparks the affair. Shared secrets—including the secrecy of the affair—may heighten the sense of having a special connection or bond. The intimacy of an affair often feels similar to the intimacy experienced early in courtship—extended passionate conversations uncomplicated by the stress of everyday life, feelings of being cared for in a special way, or special efforts to be together. You may have been drawn to your partner in part because his needs for emotional closeness matched or balanced your own, and your partner's capacity for intimacy may have helped fill your own need for emotional connection. But what started out as a shared bond may have made your partner vulnerable to an affair if your emotional connection has been disrupted.

Intimacy can be complicated. Partners need to be able to pursue emotional connection while also tolerating frustrations and separateness. If your partner has difficulty achieving this balance—either because of struggles in the relationship or because of personal limitations—he may find an affair an attractive alternative, because it appears to offer intimacy without the clutter of long-term marriage. Or the intimacy of an affair may seem to make a nonintimate marriage tolerable. If your partner is frightened by the emotional closeness and vulnerability in your marriage, an affair may appear to provide the only viable means of connecting emotionally because of its inherent limits in terms of time, expectations, and external pressures.

Ginnie's family had never been particularly close. Her parents worked hard and had little energy left at the end of the day to spend with Ginnie or her younger sister. When Ginnie first met Steve, she found his devotion comforting. But soon into their marriage she sometimes found his dependence a bit suffocating. Steve had no friends other than Ginnie, didn't seem to have any interests of his own, and resented Ginnie's desire for separate time for herself. Ginnie gradually began to pull away from Steve in order to reestablish some independence and pursue a few of her own interests. But Steve's resentment then made it more difficult to get back together to enjoy time as a couple.

In some ways, Adam seemed just the opposite of Steve. Adam had never been married, had lots of male and female friends, and pursued a life full of activities outside of work and home. He and Ginnie met while working together on a neighborhood renovation project. Soon Ginnie was leaving work early to be with Adam before Steve came home from work. Adam enjoyed Ginnie and started coming on to her early in their friendship. He didn't want any emotional commitments, which led Ginnie to believe their affair didn't need to jeopardize her marriage. Her friendship and sexual intimacy with Adam was deeply satisfying, and she found it odd that since beginning her affair with Adam she actually seemed less distant and less irritable at home.

How do you view your partner's needs for emotional connection? In what ways have these been a source of strength in the marriage, and in what ways have they been a challenge or burden? If you and your partner felt more emotionally intimate earlier in the marriage, what would it take to restore more of those feelings now?

Fulfillment of Unrealistic Expectations

No marriage—and no spouse—is perfect. Maintaining a loving relationship requires that partners accept and value each other for who they are, with all their imperfections. That doesn't mean relinquishing the right to request changes in your partner's behavior, and it doesn't mean giving in to abuse or neglect. But it does mean recognizing and coming to peace with the reality that no individual and no relationship will ever satisfy all your needs all the time. Failing to come to grips with this will ultimately bring hurt and disappointment to both partners.

Sometimes the affair partner or affair relationship provides something that's missing in the marriage. It may be passionate sex, freedom from demands or expectations, hours of snuggling or conversations free from criticism or disapproval, time away from work in exciting or relaxed settings, escape from life's hassles, and so on. The truth is that no marriage can compete with an affair on these terms. No marriage can be devoted so exclusively to mutual affirmation and pleasuring. Affairs are protected from many of the hassles, pressures, and demands of daily living that intrude into marriage. Although most partners recognize this, many still hold on to remnants of unrealistic expectations or beliefs about their marriage that can get them into trouble. Examples are:

"If our marriage is really a good one . . . " (or "If you really love me . . . "), **then:**
>   —We won't ever have serious disagreements or arguments.
>   —You'll never hurt my feelings or disappoint me.

—You'll know how I feel without my having to tell you.
—You'll always be there for me when I need you.
—We'll always place each other as our top priority.
—We'll have frequent and passionate sex.

Similarly, unrealistic expectations or beliefs about affairs can get partners into trouble. Examples include:

- As long as no one else knows about the affair, no one needs to get hurt.
- Just about everyone has affairs or wants to; they're to be expected.
- A good affair can make a bad marriage better.
- Affairs don't need to be complicated or intrude into other areas of life.

Difficulties in tolerating the inevitable disappointments that occur in a marriage, feelings of entitlement or having a sense that "I deserve better than this," and a naive lack of understanding about the limitations and frequently painful consequences of infidelity can all raise a partner's vulnerability to becoming involved in an affair. So too can the relentless pursuit of someone or something new, the excitement of seduction and engaging in a secretive liaison, the passion of a new "first kiss," and all the other heightened sensations that frequently accompany an affair.

To what extent does your partner become bored with "sameness" and require new experiences and a high level of excitement in life? Do your partner's standards for a "good marriage" seem unattainable? Could the two of you find a better way to tolerate and accept each other's limitations and imperfections, while continuing to work together toward changes in yourselves and in the marriage desired by each other?

What Did the Other Person Find in My Partner?

The same personal qualities that attracted you to your partner may cause her to be pursued by others. They, too, may find your partner particularly understanding, thoughtful, intelligent, charming, and physically attractive or sensual. Your partner may also be more desirable to others if she appears more outgoing and comfortable in discussing relationships and intimate feelings. Your partner's professional achievements, visibility in the community through public service or contributions to civic organizations, or physical fitness and attractiveness intended in part to maintain your own sexual interest may all contribute to her being emotionally or sexually attractive to others.

Does this mean your partner shouldn't work so hard to achieve success, shouldn't be as warm and caring to others, or should allow his physical appearance to go to pot? Of course not! However, it does mean he needs to recognize his social "currency" or attractiveness to others, maintain suitable vigilance, and keep his relationships with others from approaching the boundaries of inappropriate social, emotional, or physical closeness. It means your partner has to recognize flirtation and set limits on this so as not to encourage sexual advances. It means your partner must recognize when someone outside the marriage is particularly vulnerable or emotionally needy and set clear limits on his own caring to avoid promoting a level of involvement that could threaten your marriage. Your partner has to anticipate situations where interactions apart from others—as in private meetings—could promote feelings of closeness that could easily escalate. And your partner must recognize that—by virtue of his standing in the work setting, community, social group, or on the playing field—he may be a prime candidate for someone outside the marriage looking to "score" a conquest or advance in her own social status.

What positive qualities place your partner at higher risk for being sought out by someone outside your marriage? What steps would your partner need to take to recognize his or her attractiveness to others, adopt an appropriate level of vigilance, and set boundaries on interactions with others in order to protect the emotional and sexual security of your marriage?

Why Didn't My Partner Resist?

Regardless of what was going on in or around your marriage, regardless of how unhappy your partner was or how vigorously she was pursued by someone else, why didn't your partner resist? Why didn't she "just say no"? Restoring emotional security will require more than lowering vulnerabilities and attractions to an affair; it will require confidence that your partner will continue to say no to an outside relationship when things in your own marriage are at their very worst. Following are some of the factors that typically lower someone's resistance to an affair.

Problems with Commitment

It's not unusual for spouses to have times they aren't particularly happy with each other and don't "feel like" staying married, but remain faithful from a sense of obligation, responsibility, or commitment. Resolutions to remain committed can, however, be challenged by the intensity or duration of problems in the marriage and by a partner's attraction to someone else or another person's attraction to that partner. Commitment can also be undermined by despair about whether the marriage will ever get better. Feelings of desperation wouldn't excuse your partner's decision to have an affair, but they may make it less incomprehensible to you.

You need to assess your partner's capacity for commitment. Has your partner frequently been willing to set aside his own needs to accommodate someone else? If so, then his affair probably doesn't simply reflect an inability to commit. However, if your partner has a history of engaging in dishonesty or deception, or pursuit of gratification today regardless of the consequences tomorrow, problems with commitment may be an important contributing factor.

Lapses in Judgment

Related to problems with commitment are lapses in judgment— impulsive, mostly unplanned actions that are driven primarily by emotions rather than by rational thought. Some people have an impulsive style that involves only limited consideration of what's happening in the moment or what's likely to follow. They tend to act before they think and to leap before they look.

Sometimes lapses in judgment result from naivety and failure to recognize the complex or hidden motives of others. When Sheryl's art instructor offered to tutor her at his apartment at night because of "understanding" her struggles as an older student with two young children, she never imagined that he might have anything other than honorable intentions; she later was surprised by her instructor's sexual advances and found herself drawn into kissing and intimate touching before regaining her composure and putting on the brakes.

At other times, lapses in judgment relate directly to abuse of alcohol or other substances that lower inhibitions or heighten impulsivity. Similarly, impaired judgment sometimes results from emotional disorders such

as a manic–depressive or bipolar disorder. A partner's affair doesn't indicate that she has an emotional disorder. But if your partner does struggle
with an emotional disorder or with problems of substance abuse, it's important to consider how such difficulties contribute to lapses in judgment
and what steps your partner could take to lower the risks.

> Thad had a passion for life that Nita found captivating when they first
> met. He brought excitement to their relationship—an appealing con-
> trast to the tedious work and routines at home that had dominated
> her life before she met him. Thad introduced her to all kinds of
> things—rock concerts, motorcycling, "underground" movies, even
> skydiving. He had been completely open with her about his past—
> including a failed marriage—but she felt reassured by his kindness
> and genuine caring for her. When Nita eventually grew tired of partic-
> ipating in some of the adventures that Thad was drawn to, she felt al-
> most relieved when he suggested going on his own so she could have
> some quiet time for herself.
>
> When Nita learned from a mutual friend several years into their
> marriage that Thad had recently had sex with a woman he had just
> met at an out-of-town concert, her vision of Thad shattered. Al-
> though he showed deep remorse and vowed to be faithful from then
> on, Nita eventually concluded that she could never again feel secure
> in their marriage. Thad's history reflected a recurring pattern of pur-
> suing thrills and experiences that undermined his personal commit-
> ments. In the year following his affair, Thad's need for new exploits
> drew him to people and places that Nita simply wasn't comfortable
> with. After months of examining how his infidelity had come about
> and becoming clearer about aspects of Thad that he seemed unable
> or unwilling to change, Nita tearfully announced her decision to
> move on separately.

Reluctance to Confront Marital Difficulties

When a marriage suffers from significant or enduring problems, the challenge is to engage one's partner in looking at them together and trying to
resolve them as well as possible. That can involve the risk of disapproval,
being held accountable for a major portion of the problems, or having
your concerns ignored and feeling unimportant. A decision *not* to have an

affair often requires a choice between either accepting the limitations of one's partner or marriage or confronting these difficulties and working toward change. When partners feel unable to express themselves, when they fear that voicing their unhappiness may lead to further arguing, or when they're reluctant to go through the difficult process of constructive conflict, retreat to an affair can seem a safer alternative.

How able and willing is your partner to express concerns in the marriage? What would it take from both of you to create a safer and more constructive process for confronting relationship hurt and disappointment?

Expression of Discontent

Some people have an affair as a way of communicating feelings to a partner that they're having difficulty expressing more directly. The most common example is when an affair serves as a final, desperate plea to the other to "hear" that partner's profound unhappiness and need for change. The affair becomes a last-ditch effort to be heard, to gain the other partner's attention, to pronounce loudly that "we've got a major serious problem here and, unless we find a way to fix this, our marriage simply isn't going to last." Sometimes the message isn't as much a plea for collaborative change as an expression of anger. "I'm so hurt by you [or angry at you] that I can't put it into words, but I can show you by doing something that I know will hurt you just as much." The problem, of course, is that this is a high-stakes game. The message may finally be heard, but sometimes the accompanying damage is so great that healing is impossible.

Less frequently, an affair may serve not as a plea to be heard, but rather as an unspoken announcement of a decision to end the marriage. These are sometimes described as "exit" affairs. The participating partner has already reached a decision, consciously or not, to leave the marriage and anticipates that having an affair will provoke the other partner to end it for him.

You need to find out from your partner if he considered leaving the marriage when becoming involved in the affair. If so, has he changed his mind? If the affair was used in part as a means of expressing unhappiness, will your partner pledge to express these feelings directly and continue to seek your constructive engagement in the future, even when he feels discouraged about the outcome?

How Could My Partner Continue?

Thalia struggled to understand Dion's year-long affair with his best friend's wife. Dion had finally confessed to his involvement after one of their children overheard him on the phone planning another secret rendezvous. "How could you have done it?" Thalia repeatedly asked. "How could you make love to her, and then come home as though nothing had happened and make love to me?" Dion's ability to lead a dual life deeply troubled Thalia. The betrayal from the affair was traumatic enough. But how could he continue the affair and then act as though nothing was wrong? The continued deception seemed even worse than the affair. "How can I ever believe you again when you lied over and over and had me so completely fooled?"

Thalia's dilemma is a common one. A brief affair ended by the participating partner creates its own trauma. But when a partner continues involvement in an affair, maintaining the illicit relationship usually requires repeated lies that compound the trauma further. Elaborate cover stories are constructed to conceal secret trysts. Telephone bills for the cell phone used to call the other person may be sent to work or to an undisclosed post office box; separate e-mail accounts used solely for exchanges with the outside person are kept secret. Gifts for the other person are purchased in cash or with a separate credit card known only to the participating partner. Perhaps most painful of all, the participating partner may continue to be emotionally or sexually intimate with his spouse as though the outside relationship doesn't even exist. This ability to separate the outside relationship from interactions with the injured partner so completely may seem incomprehensible. "How could she have feelings for both of us and still act this way?" "How could he keep up the charade for so long?" "How can I ever trust her when she lied for so long with such ease?"

If your partner engaged in an ongoing affair, understanding both *why* and *how* he or she continued in that relationship is critical to recovery.

Why Did My Partner Continue?

Reasons your partner may have continued the outside relationship include:

• *Emotional attachment or feelings of responsibility to the outside person.* Cortney may have left her husband anyway, but Travis knew she had done so in part because of their year-long affair. Cortney was utterly alone now, and Travis just didn't feel he could abandon her while she worked through her divorce.

- **Positive aspects of the outside relationship.** Kyla found Greg easy to be with—a caring listener who appreciated her playfulness and could tolerate her occasional moodiness. The playfulness at home had faded away years ago.

- **Pessimism about the outcome of the marriage.** Ruth had expressed her concerns about their marriage as gently as she knew how, but Noah dismissed her feelings and told her she was unrealistic. When Ruth suggested marriage counseling, Noah replied "I just don't think we need that." If he wouldn't talk with her, how could things ever get better?

- **Feelings of entitlement or lack of concern about "getting caught."** Rick worked two jobs to support the family while Abby raised the kids. He didn't expect eternal gratitude, but at least she could show some appreciation and try to be a little more affectionate. He didn't want to end the marriage, but he wasn't about to go through life without sex either. He was in his prime. What did she expect?

- **Mentally separating and isolating the marriage and outside relationship.** Leah never could have imagined being unfaithful—it went against everything she believed in. But the marriage at times felt unbearable, and her escape into Sean's arms offered a different world. She never let her two worlds meet. She didn't discuss her marriage or let herself think about her family when she was with Sean, and she didn't allow herself to think of Sean when she was at home. It helped that Sean lived out of town.

Paradoxically, some of the qualities that you value in your partner may have contributed to her continuing the affair. For example, you may have been drawn to your partner in part because of her capacity to form a deep emotional and caring relationship. As hurtful as it may be to consider, it's possible that this quality contributed to a meaningful and intimate relationship with the outside person. It *is* possible to be in love with two different people at once, sometimes for different reasons and in different ways. Similarly, if your partner is someone you've viewed in the past as being responsible and honorable, it may be this sense of responsibility for the other person that contributed to maintaining the affair. Although it may seem like a distorted sense of responsibility, it's not uncommon for a participating partner to struggle with not wanting to hurt either a spouse or the outside person while feeling accountable for the well-being of both.

As couple therapists, we've worked with numerous participating partners who've struggled to end an affair, only to be drawn back in when the outside person pleads not being able to live without the participating partner or threatens to hurt him- or herself.

Of course, there also are reasons for continuing an affair that are less readily understood or forgiven. Your partner may have continued the affair simply because he could get away with it. The affair may have been exciting and gratifying, and your partner intended to maintain it so long as it continued to be rewarding and the costs related to the affair (such as time, money, or threats to the marriage) remained low. Or your partner may have continued the affair because he was preparing to leave the marriage but wasn't yet willing to tell you and deal with the consequences.

Part of what you need to assess is how much your partner struggled internally while continuing the affair. Were there times when your partner considered telling you but didn't want to hurt you or risk damaging the marriage, perhaps losing it? Did your partner ever consider or actually try ending the relationship with the other person? If you're convinced that your partner maintained the outside relationship "with ease"—that he experienced no guilt, shame, or turmoil from continued deception and betrayal—then you'll likely find it more difficult to reestablish trust and emotional security.

How Did My Partner Continue?

Beyond asking *why* your partner continued in the affair are questions about *how* your partner did so. How did she create and maintain a dual life? How could your partner continue to interact with you as though the affair relationship didn't even exist? To understand this common experience, therapists use the term *compartmentalization*—individuals' ability to take the thoughts, feelings, and behaviors of one situation and literally "shut them off as in a compartment" from their thoughts, feelings, and behaviors in a different situation.

We all engage in compartmentalization to some extent. Think about the last time you and your partner were arguing and the phone rang. Did you suspend the anger in your voice and answer the call in your usual warm and courteous manner? Or think about the last time you and your partner drove to work, church, or some social event following a bitter argument at home with each other or with one of your children. Did you mask the inner turmoil and put on your "happy face" when you walked through the door and greeted others? If your work requires you to be "on stage" or interact with others throughout the day, do you sometimes put the conflict from home aside during the day—literally out of mind—only to feel the tension reemerge at the end of the day as you're driving home?

This same process of compartmentalization is the most frequent explanation for how individuals involved in an affair maintain their dual lives. For most participating partners, an affair *does* create inner conflict. It *is* inconsistent with their values, with how they see themselves, and with their genuine caring for a spouse. Compartmentalizing the affair relationship—actually separating off the other person when with the spouse—and shutting out thoughts of their marriage when with the affair partner—is often the only way of emotionally managing the conflict.

Of course, compartmentalization implies that there's an internal struggle to be managed. Occasionally no such internal struggle exists—as when a partner's affair reflects an underlying inability to commit or to experience guilt or remorse for hurting others. Internal struggles regarding an ongoing affair also may be reduced if the participating partner has decided to leave the marriage, although sometimes a decision to end the marriage reflects an effort to manage the inner conflict resulting from an affair when compartmentalization doesn't work.

Your understanding of how your partner continued the affair will be influenced by how you viewed her character prior to the affair. Was your partner someone who generally tried to do the right thing? Did she feel bad after hurting your feelings by something she said or did? If your answer to such questions is "yes" or "most of the time," then *compartmentalization* may explain how your partner managed her own emotions while maintaining the affair and keeping it secret from you.

Why Won't My Partner End It?

If your partner is continuing the affair and doesn't want to end it, then you're likely facing all kinds of difficult decisions. Do you give your partner a deadline and an ultimatum? Do you demand a separation while the affair is going on, or do you file for divorce? Do you "wait it out" and trust that your partner will come to his senses and return to the marriage, or hope that the infatuation with the other person will burn itself out? In struggling with such questions, you may want to review material in Chapter 4 on how to respond when the affair is still going on. Your decisions about how to deal with your partner's continued involvement in an affair may depend in part on your understanding of why he is reluctant or unwilling to end it—something we'll consider further now and again in Exercise 9.2.

Positive Aspects of the Affair Relationship

Affairs provide more than pleasure. They often provide comfort, relief from life's struggles, or escape from conflicts at home. The chaos and emotional turmoil that frequently consume a marriage after an affair becomes known make it even more difficult for a marriage to compete at this time. Participating partners frequently have to choose between an affair that feels safe and comforting and a marriage that feels profoundly distressing and a partner who is hurt, angry, and demanding. Choosing the latter requires giving up something that may feel extremely good for something that may feel extremely bad. Doing so requires choosing more discomfort in the marriage in the short term in the belief that something more valuable can be restored or created in the marriage in the long term.

Emotional Connection to the Outside Person

If the affair relationship has lasted beyond a brief period, there's a good chance that your partner may have developed a deep emotional connection to the outside person. Early in affairs, unrealistic idealization of the outside person and feelings of infatuation are common. However, we've worked with participating partners whose relationship with the outside person has lasted for months or even years. In such situations, the outside relationship has often matured beyond infatuation to develop into deep knowledge of and caring for the other person. Once such a relationship has developed, it's far more difficult to end the affair. Your partner also may feel responsible for the other person's emotional well-being or feel guilty about hurting the outside person by ending the affair. We don't expect you to have much empathy for the outside person, but it may be important for you to recognize and understand what feelings your participating partner still has for the other person that could be contributing to difficulty in ending the other relationship.

> Maggie was a caretaker by nature. After her youngest child left home, her life felt empty. Her husband, Russ, was a faithful provider but didn't seem to need much emotionally from their marriage. Mag-

gie met Delsin after she began volunteering at her community's hospice program. Delsin was recently widowed and utterly adrift. Weekly lunches with Maggie quickly became the high point in his life. Maggie felt drawn to Delsin not only because of his gentle and kind nature, but also because of his obvious deep need for her emotionally. It felt so good to be needed. When she and Delsin first made love several months after first meeting, for Maggie it wasn't at all about the sex. It was about giving in a deeply intimate way to someone who just melted into her arms.

Russ learned of the affair from a friend who had seen Maggie leaving Delsin's home. He insisted she sever her relationship with Delsin immediately, and Maggie agreed. But her promise proved difficult to keep. Delsin e-mailed her daily, professing how deeply he loved Maggie and needed her. He was desperate and just couldn't bear another loss like this. He needed at least to see her. Maggie consented, and several secret meetings followed. There was no further lovemaking, but Maggie found herself needing their emotional connection as much as Delsin. With Russ being so hurt and angry with her, the aloneness at home felt unbearable.

Pessimism about the Outcome of the Marriage

Your partner's reluctance to give up the affair may also be influenced by ongoing difficulties or current chaos in your own relationship and pessimism or despair about things ever getting better. If long-standing struggles in the marriage contributed to your partner's initial vulnerability to an affair, these conflicts may make it more difficult to commit to the marriage now. Your partner may also be assessing the future quality of your marriage by predicting from the current emotional turmoil rather than considering previous times in your marriage that were less chaotic and more satisfying.

What hopefulness does your partner express about your ability to move beyond this trauma together? Does she recount times in the past when things were significantly better? Can you communicate your own hopefulness for how you can restore or create a better marriage for both of you?

Inability or Unwillingness to Commit to One Person

Your partner may not want to commit to a monogamous relationship with you. Or he may be willing to end the sexual aspects of an outside relationship but insist on the right to continue a close relationship with the outside affair person on a nonsexual level. Alternatively, your partner may verbally commit to an emotionally and sexually exclusive relationship with you, but continue to be vulnerable to outside relationships because of excessive needs for affirmation, lapses in judgment, or inability to defer his own gratification for the sake of the marriage. In addition to evaluating how your partner became involved in the affair in the first place, if the affair is continuing, you'll need to assess your partner's capacity for commitment.

Why Can't My Partner Move On?

Once an affair has ended, moving on requires that you and your partner work through the trauma of the affair and collaborate in understanding how it came about. It also requires that eventually you both allow thoughts and feelings about the affair to recede into the background as you work toward the future together. Your partner may have difficulty with any of these steps.

Working Through the Trauma

You and your partner may continue to struggle with the challenges described in Part I of this book. Participating partners often recognize how hurt the injured partner continues to be and fear any discussion that dredges up these hurt feelings. Part of their reluctance to engage in discussions about the affair may stem from the chaos of stirring things up all over again. Does your partner feel "worn down" by the continued turmoil in your marriage? How can you work together to make discussions about the affair less traumatic for you both?

Your partner may also be wrestling with difficult feelings of his own. For example, he may be struggling with having ended a close emotional connection to the outside person, but also recognizes how difficult it might be for you to hear those feelings. Other times participating partners wrestle with their own frustrations regarding their marriages but don't believe they're entitled to express such feelings because of what they've done in having an affair.

Try talking with your partner about his or her reluctance to discuss the affair. What's making it difficult?

Understanding How the Affair Came About

Participating partners sometimes find it difficult to explore how an affair came about because they're literally confused and overwhelmed themselves about why the affair happened. Your partner may not be able to recognize or label the feelings he was having toward you, your marriage, or the outside person that contributed to the affair. Or your partner may have difficulty expressing those feelings to you without becoming overwhelmed by the intensity of your feelings or reactions to her explanations.

> *Palomi described her frustration in trying to talk with her husband, Kavi, about the reasons for her affair. "He says he wants to know what drove me to it, but he really doesn't. When I talk about how lonely and desperate I felt, he responds by saying, 'How do you think I feel now?' Then Kavi tells me that I wasn't any dream partner, and he still didn't cheat on me. I know I've hurt him deeply, but trying to talk about what was missing in our marriage just seems to hurt him more."*

Your partner's motive for *not* wanting to discuss the affair may be to protect you from further hurt or disappointment. Or your partner may be convinced that everything that can be said has already been said. Your questions may seem repetitive and unanswerable. Think about discussions you and your partner have had about why the affair occurred. Do you seem stuck in going over and over the same questions, mostly getting the same answers? What would you or your partner consider a sign of progress in these discussions?

Moving from Thoughts and Feelings Rooted in the Past

Your partner may be reluctant to "forget what happened," just as you may be. Some participating partners believe that an important safeguard against "slipping up" in the future is to remind themselves constantly about how they've "messed up" in the past. As therapists, we don't encourage participating partners to forget the affair, but we do advise them against being consumed endlessly about thoughts of the affair and reeling in guilt. At some point, guilt loses its effectiveness as a motivator and becomes a barrier to intimacy.

You may have initially found your partner's guilt reassuring as a safeguard against future betrayal, but subsequently found that your partner's preoccupation with the affair prevents your moving on together. If so, talk with your partner about what you need now in the relationship and how that differs from what you needed after you first learned of the affair. How do you want the two of you to rediscover joy and spontaneity? What are you able to contribute to that effort now that you couldn't earlier?

Creating a Future Together

You and your partner won't be able to work toward creating a better future together unless you share at least some hopefulness that such a future is possible. Once the affair has ended, your partner's pessimism regarding the marriage may continue to block efforts to work together toward building or restoring a more satisfying marriage. If you find yourself in this position, talk with your partner about why you need him to join with you in working through the healing process and rebuilding your marriage. Talk about the advantages you envision for both of you in working through this together and your confidence in your ability to do so. If your own pessimism has discouraged your partner from working toward a future together, what would it take to challenge your pessimism and promote feelings of hopefulness for both of you?

> Becky, whose husband Nick we described at the beginning of this chapter, struggled to make sense of her husband's affair. If nothing else, Nick had always been someone she could count on. From the earliest days of their relationship he had been sensitive and caring and committed to Becky's well-being and, later, the well-being of their children. Nick was a good, honest person, and she loved him deeply.
>
> In the months after Nick disclosed his affair, he and Becky talked about the distance that had gradually grown between them as Nick's success with the company drew him away from home and Becky's involvement with the children sometimes kept her from being with him. Nick was reluctant to complain about any of the shortcomings in

their marriage, because he deeply admired all Becky had done for him and their children. Although profoundly hurt by Nick's affair, Becky eventually persuaded him that she cared less about "fault" for the distance that had developed in their marriage and cared more about finding ways to overcome it.

Nick struggled with his remorse and shame in having betrayed Becky. He was reluctant to examine any explanations that might make it "easier" to understand, because he explicitly did not want it to be "easy" for him. But gradually Nick struggled through his guilt to confront long-standing issues involving his own lingering self-doubts that had their roots back in adolescence. He and Diana, the woman with whom he had the affair, had gone to school together. She had always been one of those women that he considered "beyond his reach." Nick had to confront the demons of his self-doubts and shed these before he could fully embrace the goodness and completeness of his relationship with Becky.

Becky didn't simply "get over" Nick's affair after developing a better understanding of his needs that had contributed to it. She continued to hurt. But Nick's affair became less terrifying to her, less like a random act that could repeat itself, and less like a response to something fundamentally wrong about herself. By examining the aspects of himself that had contributed to his affair, Nick also seemed better able to understand what had happened as a way of making sure it didn't happen again. He could now recognize his occasional feelings of loneliness in the marriage more easily, and he learned to express these in ways that helped Becky feel needed rather than criticized, and for both of them to regain the closeness they each desired rather than drifting farther apart.

What's Next?

Complete the following exercises. If you and your partner are both working through these chapters, do the exercises separately but then arrange a time to compare and discuss your responses. Then move on to Chapter 10, where we'll encourage you to consider the roles you played in your marriage prior to the affair, as a way of understanding the larger context in which your partner's affair occurred.

Exercises

EXERCISE 9.1. ASPECTS OF THE PARTICIPATING PARTNER CONTRIBUTING TO THE AFFAIR

Whether you're the injured or the participating partner, you both need to take an honest look at the person who had the affair. What characteristics made this person vulnerable to an affair? Some of these factors may have been present for a long time—for example, turning to other people for attention and affection when the relationship wasn't going well. Other factors might be more recent or short-lived, such as uncharacteristic poor judgments while under unusual pressure at work. In examining aspects of the participating partner, it's important to be honest and balanced. If there are difficult things to confront, now is the time to do so. At the same time, don't portray the participating partner in exaggerated negative ways, even if that makes it easier to explain what happened. In fact, some of these factors that made the person vulnerable might actually be positive qualities that were handled badly. Understanding both negative and positive characteristics of the participating partner that potentially contributed to the affair can help both of you understand what would need to change and whether you believe your relationship can endure.

List the major factors about the participating partner that made him or her vulnerable to an affair. What was the participating partner looking for in the affair, and was this unusual or more typical for this person? For example, perhaps you believe that the participating partner typically likes to feel close to people of the opposite sex and encourages that closeness in ways that put your relationship at risk. Or the participating partner might have experienced a major disappointment at work or at home and was feeling particularly uncertain about his or her self-worth. Which aspects of the participating partner contributing to vulnerability to an affair have been present for a long time, and which ones have developed more recently?

EXERCISE 9.2. ASPECTS OF THE PARTICIPATING PARTNER THAT HELP OR HINDER RECOVERY

There might be aspects of the participating partner that make it more difficult to recover from the affair or make that person more vulnerable to affairs in the future. For example, you might believe that your partner has always avoided dealing with problems in the marriage, and now doesn't seem willing to face how destructive the affair was, either:

"If she won't face obvious conflicts right in front of her, how will we ever recover from this horrible experience?"

Or you might believe that your partner was allowed to have whatever he or she wanted when growing up, and this continuing expectation in your relationship contributed to the affair:

"If his long-term attitude doesn't change, will he have another affair if he finds someone attractive again in the future?"

Likewise, the participating partner may have real strengths and qualities that offer promise for a secure future together. For example, you may conclude that when this person has made a major mistake in the past, he or she has typically accepted responsibility, figured out what needed to change, and then committed to make these changes, no matter how difficult. Or perhaps since the affair, the participating partner has already undertaken major changes to reduce risk factors the two of you have identified and has sustained these efforts for several months.

Make two lists. First, list characteristics of the participating partner that might make recovery from the affair difficult or make this person vulnerable to an affair in the future. Second, list strengths or positive qualities of the participating partner that might help in recovery from the affair or protect you from an affair in the future.

────────────────────────

10

What Was My Role?

When Brenda first heard that Matt had been seen having dinner at an upscale restaurant with an old girlfriend, she simply didn't believe it. Brenda brought up the rumor with Matt anyway, and he denied it but promised to avoid any situations that could contribute to the stories that sometimes circulated.

That was two months ago. Then yesterday Brenda's best friend, Tanya, approached her with obvious discomfort and told Brenda about three different occasions when Matt had been seen having dinner with the same woman. Tanya didn't want to hurt Brenda, but said that she also felt uncomfortable knowing something hurtful that Brenda obviously did not. When Brenda approached Matt with the new information, he stammered and offered lame explanations. When she persisted, he finally acknowledged that he had run into his old flame six months ago, and they had been intimate several times since.

Brenda's head had been spinning and her heart pounding ever since. How could she have been so naive and not seen it coming? Sure, she and Matt had been having some pretty difficult times over the past year—she wanted children; he wasn't ready. She wanted to advance in her firm with an out-of-state move; he wanted to stay put. But she never anticipated it could lead to this. Brenda had been so angry last night that she yelled at Matt to get out of the house and vowed to call a lawyer the next day. Matt stayed at a friend's house, but Brenda didn't call an attorney. She didn't know what she wanted.

And what did Matt want to do about the marriage now? He said he still loved Brenda, but added that he had been miserable for over a year. She had chalked it up to "working out the kinks" in a young marriage and thought it was just a difficult phase that would pass. Matt apparently feared otherwise.

What did Matt want from her? He said he needed more closeness—but felt pushed away by her. He complained that she never approached him passionately, but only criticized him when she thought he had messed up somehow with their finances or forgot to do something she had asked. "You're not being fair," Brenda had told him. "How am I supposed to pour myself into my job and compete in an office dominated by men and then have enough energy left over to be passionate with you? We agreed if we were going to delay kids that this was the time to push ahead in our careers. Just be patient—we'll have more time for each other in another year or two."

Matt didn't think he could wait a couple of years, and Brenda's vision about how they would rekindle their closeness and start a family had now evaporated. Had she been wrong? Had she been blind? Was she to blame for Matt's affair? Could she get Matt back—and did she even want to try?

Brenda wasn't responsible for Matt's decision to have an affair—no matter how inattentive, tired, or critical she may have been. Matt could have been clearer with Brenda about how unhappy or even desperate he felt. He could have asked her what she needed from him so she could be available. He could have suggested they get outside help—perhaps from their minister or a marriage counselor. Matt had a choice in whether to respond to his distress by getting involved with someone else.

In no way was Brenda responsible for Matt's affair. But once she decided to consider whether their marriage could be salvaged, she needed to evaluate her own role in increasing their relationship's vulnerability to infidelity—just as the two of them had to explore Matt's role, what was going on in their marriage to begin with, and how outside influences made things worse. Brenda didn't have to agree with Matt's views of her and the marriage, but she at least needed to understand what his views were.

The main goal of this chapter is to help you, the injured partner, look at your role, but we strongly suggest that the participating partner read it too, particularly "A Special Message to the Participating Partner" on page 234, to understand both *why* and *how* to help you with the task at hand.

The work we're encouraging you to do in this chapter is very difficult. If you've asked your partner how he or she could have betrayed you like this, your partner may have tried to assure you that there was nothing wrong with the marriage. We're asking you to step back and ask yourself now whether you believe this. We want you to think about what you could have done to make the marriage stronger, knowing what you know now. What was going on within you or in the world around you that made it difficult for you to be the kind of partner you'd really like to be? If you think you may want to restore your marriage, what would that require of you right now—as well as six months or a year from now?

If just reading these questions brings up all the hurt and anger you felt right after the affair came to light, you may not be ready to do some of this work. In that case, read through Chapter 6 again to see whether you can find your way to a different perspective. It may help to remember that *reasons* for an affair are never *excuses* and that *understanding* your partner's perspective isn't the same as *agreeing* with it. Moreover, we've said it several times, but it bears repeating: Even if you decide not to stay in this marriage, taking a close look at yourself and understanding yourself better may help you achieve greater intimacy and security in future relationships.

In this chapter, we'll encourage you first to consider what roles you played in the marriage prior to your partner's affair. Then we'll ask you to examine your roles in the marriage during and following the affair.

A Special Message to the Participating Partner

As the participating partner who had the affair, you have two critical roles in this particular part of the recovery process. First, you have unique information that your partner needs and can get only from you. Only you know what vital positive elements in your marriage may have felt lacking, or what negative qualities gradually eroded your feelings of closeness or hopefulness for the future. It's also possible that you were quite happy with your partner and that the vulnerabilities in your marriage weren't the critical factors that led to your having an affair. But given that the affair occurred and you want to move forward, both of you now need to explore whether your partner contributed to any vulnerabilities in your marriage. You and your partner can't go back to the way things were; now you have to make things better.

Second, you need to recognize that your partner can't pursue this important part of understanding and recovering from the affair unless you make this process emotionally safe.

>>> **Doing so involves:**
- **Taking responsibility for your affair, regardless of what was going on in your marriage or elsewhere.**
- **Emphasizing that the goal of exploring your partner's role isn't to assign blame but to clarify what it would now take to build a better, stronger relationship together.**
- **Being sensitive to your partner's deep hurt and fears about the future of your marriage. Being sensitive means expressing your frustrations or disappointments in language that doesn't attack or overwhelm your partner.**
- **Being patient when your partner initially responds in an angry or defensive manner, and waiting for another time to continue your conversations.**

In our experience, participating partners can thwart this phase of the recovery process by going to one of two extremes. Sometimes they jump at the opportunity to examine the injured partner's role and end up blaming the partner or the marriage unfairly to excuse their own role. Obviously, this is self-defeating and will only make matters worse. Other times they resist focusing on the partner's role at all, because they're afraid it will just hurt the injured partner further, they don't want to be seen as avoiding responsibility or shifting the blame, and maybe they even feel that nothing will make the marriage better. This last prophecy is self-fulfilling: If you won't admit the possibility of improvement, and you're unwilling to take the risk of working to make things better, the marriage *can't and won't* get better. As couple therapists, we've seen that *relationship traumas such as affairs can often promote important changes in both partners that may not have been possible before.*

If you're willing but the injured partner isn't, you may be able to facilitate this discussion by reviewing the guidelines in Chapter 6. Talk with your partner about why this is important to you and emphasize what you hope will come from this process for both of you. If your partner isn't yet ready to explore the questions in this chapter, express your willingness to wait, as well as your hope that you can do this together in the near future. Then read through this chapter on your own.

Was the Affair My Fault?

If we haven't made this clear yet, the answer is an unqualified no. But could you have contributed to putting your marriage at risk of infidelity? Possibly. About half of the men and a third of the women who have an affair report that they were happily married at the time. Some may in fact have had a strong marriage, but others may answer that they were happily married by default—because they simply couldn't put a finger on anything that seemed to make their marriage vulnerable to an affair. Others may report being "happily married" despite significant shortcomings in the marriage because they want to protect the partner or because they're reluctant to consider what it would require to improve it. Asserting "it's me—not you" can sometimes be a misguided gesture of caring or a way of avoiding important change.

Whether your goal at this moment is to save this marriage or to ensure that you're not vulnerable to the same trauma in any future relationship, you need to consider what you bring to a relationship that may prevent your marriage from working as well as you'd like. As you read the following pages and work through Exercise 10.1, think about the ways in which people sometimes make their relationship vulnerable to an affair, including the following obstacles:

- Difficulties in meeting your partner's needs for intimacy or for personal growth.
- Unrealistic expectations or demands.
- Negative behaviors that were too frequent or intense.
- Difficulty in recovering from relationship disappointments or conflicts.
- Difficulty in dealing with differences in styles of thinking and feeling.
- Reluctance to work on your own contributions to relationship difficulties.

Did I Fail to Meet My Partner's Needs?

You can't possibly fulfill all of your partner's wishes or desires. All you can hope for is that you'll strive to meet each other's needs as well as possible to care for one another and nurture your marriage. In Chapter 7 we described a number of qualities that are important to most marriages—

emotional connectedness, physical intimacy, and opportunities for personal growth and fulfillment. Knowing what you know now about your partner and about how healthy marriages work, are there ways you could have made the marriage better?

Consider your emotional relationship. How important have emotional connection and intimacy been to you and your partner throughout your marriage? Think back to times when your partner may have wanted simply to relax or play together but you thought it was more important to get some work done. Did creating opportunities to be together become primarily your partner's responsibility—so that your partner no longer felt pursued by you? Was physical intimacy lacking in any way? Did your partner prefer a different kind of physical intimacy than you did, such as more nonsexual touching?

Finally, reflect on your partner's needs to grow as an individual. Did you listen to your partner's frustrations and dreams, supporting your partner in good times and bad? If despite your best intentions and efforts, you sometimes fell short in fostering intimacy and personal growth, what would you be willing to do differently?

> *After Mayra's mother died, an emptiness washed over her that she couldn't shake; her children were off having families of their own, and her husband, Carlos, seemed absorbed in managing his thriving orthopedics practice. Carlos recognized that Mayra was struggling, but he wasn't sure how to respond. Mayra had always been fiercely independent. He would never have expected her to feel desperate enough to succumb to an affair.*

Did I Drive My Partner Away?

You didn't drive your partner to having an affair. But you may have contributed to hurtful exchanges or permitted stressors from the outside to have a destructive impact. How would your partner describe your approach to dealing with differences between the two of you? Think of times when your partner was clearly upset; were you able to acknowledge his feelings without responding with your own complaints? Or when your own feelings were hurt, were you able to address these in a constructive way? In addition to resolving disagreements, did you both do what was needed to protect your marriage from outside stressors? Try to identify what you would need to do differently now to keep outside influences from affecting your marriage negatively and to give your relationship a higher priority.

What expectations of your own did you bring into your relationship? Although having high expectations for your family can be a good thing, *excessive* expectations or demands can fuel resentment or cause your partner to believe that whatever she does will never be good enough. What did you want from your marriage? How did you communicate these needs and desires, and did your partner feel able to meet these expectations?

> *Trudy and Logan had known each other since the seventh grade and married two years into college, but then their paths started to diverge. She entered veterinary school, while he took over a portion of his family's ranch. Trudy was disappointed that Logan lacked ambition and seemed content to live out a quiet, modest life as his parents had. She wanted more for them and encouraged Logan to take courses through the college extension service and pursue partnerships in neighboring ranches that were becoming available. The more she pushed, the deeper he dug in. When Trudy's clinic responsibilities drew her away at night and she seemed passionless during infrequent lovemaking, Logan felt progressively less desired and less valued. Within a year, he pursued an affair with a woman he had known in college.*

What Did the Outside Person Have That I Don't?

There may be a variety of things that the outside affair person had that you don't, but we want to be clear about one that stands out above all the rest: *The outside affair person had the luxury of interacting with your partner in a relationship that was devoted exclusively to mutual pleasure, without all the additional responsibilities and intrusions that confront a marriage.* This, more than anything else, defines the fundamental difference between an affair and a marriage. It also accounts for why you can't compete in the same ways with an affair partner. You have different roles. We emphasize this point to make sure that neither you nor your partner compares you with the outside person in ways that are simply unrealistic and unfair.

Of course, the other person may have additional positive characteristics that you can't realistically match. For example, you can't be five or ten years younger. You can't choose your body type, and there may be limits to your influence over your own health or other physical characteristics. You may not be able to match either the career status or the income of the outside person. You may not be able to achieve the same flexibility in your schedule or freedom from competing responsibilities. You may not always be able to look your best, put on a happy face, avoid difficult topics, express admiration for your partner, or create separate space when either you or your partner feels pressured.

By their very nature, affairs differ so dramatically from committed cohabiting or married relationships that comparing the two to determine which seems better in the long run isn't realistic. Similarly, the roles of an outside affair person and a marriage partner are so different that comparing yourself (or your partner) with the outside person is neither realistic nor productive.

How Should I Work to Be Different?

There's probably none of us who couldn't be a better partner by being more conscientious, more patient, more attentive, or more understanding. The goal in examining your contributions to the marriage isn't to work toward change from a basis of fear or guilt. Instead, the goal is to engage in a thoughtful reflection on what you value in marriage, consider how you believe loving partners can best care for each other and nurture their relationship, and carefully assess your own contributions to determine how you could come closer to being the kind of loving partner you aspire to be. Listen to your partner's concerns about your marriage and include this perspective in your assessment—but also examine your own vision for how good marriages work and what this requires on your part.

Consider also how you came to have your values and expectations regarding relationships. For example, how did you develop your own ways of dealing with difficult feelings, communicating your needs, and connecting emotionally or physically? How did your parents express their feelings toward each other and resolve conflicts or reach decisions together? Did members of your family generally "do their own thing" independently of one another? Understanding your own relationship patterns as they've developed over your lifetime may offer you a different perspective on what you'd like to keep doing in your current relationship and what you'd want to change for your own sake or for the sake of your marriage. It can also give you and your partner a sense of why you both made the choices you did in the past, as well as giving you more control over what you decide to do in the future.

Finally, be sure to keep in mind the principle of balance. Any personal characteristic, taken to the extreme, may not serve you or your relationship well. Strengths can sometimes become problematic. For example, your enduring optimism may at times have prevented you from recognizing important problems emerging in your marriage. Your deep sense of responsibility to others—your children, extended family, friends, or community—may at times have left you with little physical or emotional energy for your marriage. Your ambition and need to achieve may have interfered with the need to relax or play with your partner. Your ability and preference to think logically about issues may have blocked you at times from empathizing with your partner around important feelings.

When deciding how to work toward being a better partner, try to focus not only on limitations or shortcomings that you want to overcome but on your strengths as well and how to use them more effectively for the sake of your marriage.

Seth's friends advised him to kick Jill out of the house following her affair. How was he supposed to do that? Despite reeling in shock and anger, he really didn't want to lose Jill. Jill claimed she didn't want to lose Seth, either. She said they had drifted so far apart that she had felt as though she was drowning without a lifeline and that Seth had simply turned away.

Seth and Jill both worked 12-hour days, sometimes for weeks on end. They thrived on challenges and made a good team. They weren't sure they wanted children, but they had a few more years before needing to decide. But following Seth's last promotion, things changed. Seth vaguely recalled Jill complaining about feeling stuck in her own career and resentful of long hours with little advancement, and then being upset when Seth worked during weekends at home to finish reports. What did she expect? He was struggling with a new job himself.

Jill didn't blame Seth for her affair; she regretted that decision more deeply than she could ever express. She begged Seth to forgive her, but also to work with her to make things right. Their life was different—and what worked earlier in the marriage wasn't working anymore. Seth recognized that, for both of them, the changes would require more than minor adjustments. He didn't want Jill and himself simply to "hang on" for the next five years. If he wanted the marriage to work, they'd both have to restructure their lives in some major ways. Parts of that seemed scary, but the alternative was more terrify-ing. Seth hadn't retreated from challenges in the past, and he wasn't about to retreat from this one.

Should I Have Seen It Coming?

Intimate relationships are built in part on trust. One of the reasons that learning of a partner's affair feels so traumatic is because frequently it is so totally unexpected. You may be crying out now, "How could I have been so foolish to trust my partner? How could I have been so stupid?" There's nothing foolish or stupid about having trust. Trust in marriage is more than a "good" thing—it's essential to security and emotional intimacy.

At the same time, you may have failed to detect clear signals regard-ing your partner's unhappiness or wavering commitment in the marriage. We're not talking here about evidence that might have been uncovered if you'd been more suspicious and either taken on the role of a detective or actually hired a private investigator. Instead, we're talking specifically about situations when partners have expressed deep pessimism or disillu-sionment in the marriage, have made statements about ending the mar-riage or finding someone else if the marriage doesn't improve, or have otherwise demonstrated disregard for important expectations in the cur-rent relationship. The question to ask yourself isn't "Could I have known about the affair earlier if I had been more suspicious?" but "Were there clear signs that I could have responded to earlier to reduce the risk of an affair?"

Such "clear signs" might include, for example, that your partner stops inviting you to social events you had previously attended together—to separate you from the outside affair person or from others who may know of the affair. Some people stop providing information about how they can be reached when away—whether for the evening or when out of town. Were there other signs in your marriage? Did your partner express unhap-piness in your relationship and try unsuccessfully to get you to talk about this? Did you notice withdrawal from physical connection—for example, pulling away from your touches or no longer showing an interest in love-making?

If you can now see that the signs were there, consider what it was about yourself that might have made it more difficult either to identify or talk about these difficult aspects of your marriage. For example, perhaps your partner's unhappiness made you too nervous to talk about the issues directly, or perhaps you underestimated the problems in your marriage. Did you fail to take your partner's unhappiness seriously, believing it to be a stage that would pass with time?

Knowing what you know now, take some time to reflect on what it would take for you to be vigilant in your marriage in a healthy way—not unduly suspicious and mistrustful—but alert to early signs of relationship problems that you could address with your partner.

Could I Have Stopped It?

If someone is determined to have an affair, there's probably little that his or her partner can do to prevent it. Just as you weren't responsible for your partner's decision to have an affair, you may not have been able to prevent it or to stop it once it occurred. However, there may have been things that you did or didn't do that made the affair easier to occur, easier to continue, or more difficult to stop.

Did I Make the Affair Too Easy?

Healthy relationships have boundaries—places where you and your partner both put up a stop sign, and neither of you goes beyond that point. Such boundaries involve expectations about how you interact with each other and with those outside your relationship, including children, extended family members, friends, and coworkers. A marriage can become more vulnerable to an affair when expectations regarding relationship boundaries aren't made clear or when violations are minimized or ignored. It's possible to become too *accommodating* to your partner's behaviors that cross the line—ignoring hugs with another person that last too long, for example, or laughing at sexually oriented teasing between your partner and another person. When your partner starts to go beyond the boundaries and doesn't take personal responsibility for ending such violations, it's important for you to step in, express concern, and help to reestablish the boundaries.

People sometimes fail to realize how important such limits are—particularly if they grew up in families lacking appropriate boundaries. Were appropriate boundaries established and respected in your own family? Perhaps your parents talked about things in front of their children that should have been just between them, or people walked around the house dressed inappropriately, so that it never became clear what levels of physical display between people were appropriate. Were the boundaries between members of your family and outsiders clear and appropriate? Do you recall ever seeing either of your parents express too much affection toward other people? Do you remember times they divulged too many details about personal or family matters with people outside the family? It is mainly within families that individuals learn where to set boundaries. If your family conveyed this poorly, it might be difficult for you to know where to set boundaries in your marriage and how to evaluate them.

You may be well aware of what appropriate boundaries look like. But when you first observed them being crossed, you possibly didn't know just what to do. Many people deny or minimize the early warning signs of an affair because these signs make them so uncomfortable. Talking about them brings them out in the open and makes them more real, and you may not have wanted to risk further shattering your already shaky sense of security. You might have worried that bringing up your concerns would drive your partner into the relationship you suspected was developing. Or perhaps you feared being labeled "jealous" or immature or so insecure that you couldn't let your partner have any friends.

Avoiding difficult discussions about relationship boundaries can reduce discomfort in the short run, but runs the risk of making the marriage more vulnerable to an affair in the long run. Did you and your partner have clear agreements regarding emotionally intimate, flirtatious, or sexual interactions with others? If you observed times when your partner's behavior appeared inconsistent with such agreements, did you raise this concern directly?

Carla didn't like the way Jabari joked with other women. He did it in restaurants, at parties, at work—even at church. When she told Jabari she was uncomfortable with some of these interactions, he called her a "prude." Carla wondered whether he might be right. She had never been particularly comfortable in social gatherings, and Jabari's charming and flirtatious style was one of the qualities she had found attractive. Now she found it unsettling but kept quiet because whenever she challenged him he laughed at her for being too "uptight." Later, after learning of Jabari's affair, Carla felt foolish for having ingored her instincts and was determined to require more appropriate and respectful behavior.

Even though you now know that your partner did in fact have an affair, you might be tempted to look the other way when you see the same signs, indicating that the affair is still going on or a new one may be starting. Placing tighter limits on your partner, you might fear, will make the marriage feel more confining and an affair seem like a relief. There are all kinds of reasons that people decide not to confront an ongoing affair—to try to hold on to their marriage, preserve their own self-esteem, shelter their children from learning of the participating parent's infidelity, maintain the façade of "a happy couple" with friends and family. If your partner is continuing interactions with an outside affair person, review Chapter 4 to remind yourself of how to erect boundaries that will protect you and, where feasible and desirable, your marriage.

Did I Make the Affair More Difficult to Stop?

This is a tricky question to ask yourself. It's almost inevitable—and certainly understandable—that your interactions with your partner will be intensely negative or even punishing right after the affair has been revealed. But if intensely negative interactions continue for months or even years and the marriage no longer seems salvageable, your partner may decide that the marriage isn't worth any effort. When your partner has recently had—or is still having—an affair, it's hardly fair to insist that you relinquish any further hurt or angry behavior and instead focus only on positive interactions. But when smoldering resentment or hostile interactions persist for too long, either partner may become so discouraged and hopeless that there's little motivation for working on the marriage. Unfortunately, it's not unusual for a person having an affair to seek refuge and comfort from the outside person to escape from the hurt and anger of the injured partner.

> When Mandy discovered Lance was having an affair with Gretchen—a friend of theirs from the school board—she was furious and determined to make Lance hurt as much as she did. She told him to move out of the house, and when he balked, she insisted he sleep on a mattress thrown on the floor of the family room. When her teenage children asked what was going on, she told them everything she knew about their father's affair. Mandy called the president of the school board and insisted that Gretchen and Lance be put on separate committees. She wept bitterly to her own extended family and

made sure Lance's family knew all about Gretchen as well. Mandy suspended standing engagements with their couple friends, explaining that Lance had "become involved with someone else." Within a week, Lance had virtually no one to talk to and few places he could go without embarrassment. Even his colleagues at work knew about his affair.

Two months later little had changed. Lance had ended all contact with Gretchen and informed Mandy of this, but it made no difference. Lance knew she had already consulted an attorney. Mandy barely acknowledged him when they were together in the house. He had long since given up on having dinners with the family, staying at work after hours and picking up a sandwich before heading home. When Gretchen sent him a brief e-mail one afternoon, asking him if he was okay, Lance replied with how miserable he was. Their e-mail exchanges soon took on the same frequency and emotional depth they had had during the affair. Several weeks later, Lance and Gretchen resumed their affair.

If Mandy had thought about her reactions, she may have realized that she was giving Lance nowhere else to turn and this wasn't at all what she wanted. If you want your marriage to have a chance to recover—even if you're uncertain right now whether that's what you want in the long term—think about how frequently and how intensely you express your hurt and anger to your partner. How could you temporarily step back to help you regain control of your feelings? How do fear and profound sadness overwhelm your ability to interact with your partner in a more constructive manner? It's natural to feel deeply hurt, anxious, or angry after learning of a partner's affair, but ultimately it's important to find ways to limit or step back from these feelings.

Am I Making Recovery More Difficult?

Intense negativity and the absence of positive interactions not only can make it more difficult for your partner to end an affair, but also can make it more difficult for either of you to recover long after an affair is over. If your partner's affair has ended but you seem stuck in angry exchanges, cycling over and over through the same painful discussions without gaining any headway or relief, it's important to figure out how to try to move forward. Maybe your partner is continuing to behave in ways that threaten the security of your marriage. Or perhaps other unresolved problems in the marriage are keeping you and your partner in heightened conflict. However, it's also possible that what's going on with *you* is making recovery more difficult for either you or your partner. It's important to explore whether that's the case and, if so, how you could manage things differently. Exercise 10.2 will help you do this.

What's Making This More Difficult for Me Now?

Above and beyond the traumatic impact of a partner's affair, there may be aspects of yourself that make the initial devastation even worse than it might be otherwise, or more difficult to recover from in the weeks or months that follow. Understanding these aspects better may help you in your own recovery and may also help your partner to be more patient as you struggle to get through this.

Fear of Vulnerability

You may be finding recovery especially difficult because at some level you're still reeling from shock. The more trusting you were of your partner prior to the affair, or the harder it seemed to even *imagine* the possibility of your partner being unfaithful, the more profound the trauma of learning about the affair is likely to have been. *Recovery requires moving from exclaiming, "I can't believe it," to declaring, "I need to understand it."*

The trauma of an affair can also be worse if it reopens old wounds that never healed. These injuries might have occurred earlier in this marriage, in previous relationships, or even in the family in which you grew up. Repeated betrayals, even those experienced in different relationships, can deepen your vulnerability, magnify the intensity of hurt and anger, and fuel despair about ever having a secure and intimate relationship deserving of your trust and your heart. They can leave you struggling with the terror of allowing yourself to become vulnerable once again. The only way to remain safe for sure is to remain emotionally distant—either through conflict or by physical withdrawal. By contrast, rebuilding trust requires accepting risk; restoring intimacy demands your vulnerability. If one of the barriers to restoring closeness now involves betrayals from long ago, let your partner know this. Doing so may help both of you place the affair in a larger context in ways that allow you to be less reactive to each other.

Moral Conviction

Strong values are generally good for both individuals and relationships. But when your partner fundamentally violates a core value like commitment to emotional and sexual fidelity, it can be easy to view all of him through the lens of that violation. It can be difficult to piece together positive and negative qualities of your partner into one complete picture that makes sense. "How could I ever respect and admire someone who has done such a terrible thing?"

Sometimes a person whose partner had an affair will say, "I swore that I would never stay married to anybody who cheated on me. To go back on that now would mean I don't believe in the sanctity of marriage." The problem with this stance is that sometimes situations relate to multiple values that don't necessarily lead to the same conclusion. Some people choose to remain in marriages that are consistently destructive to themselves or their children because they value their pledge "to have and to hold, for better or worse, until death parts us." Others struggle with how to pull together their competing values affirming the importance of sexual fidelity and those affirming the importance of reconciliation and forgiveness.

We don't presume to tell you what values you should have or what priorities you should give them. But we do encourage you to consider whether you sometimes reach decisions based mostly on one particular value while ignoring others. Is it possible for you to love someone who has hurt you badly? If you value repair and recovery in intimate relationships, how can you include that value in decisions you're wrestling with about your marriage and your partner now?

Pride and Influence from Others

No one wants to appear foolish. Deciding to work toward recovery in a marriage following a partner's affair is hard enough—but it can be even more difficult if others outside the marriage send the message that doing so is "weak," "foolish," or "a big mistake." Men who continue to work on a marriage after a partner has had an affair sometimes worry that they won't appear strong or masculine to other men. Similarly, women who continue to work on a marriage after a partner's affair sometimes are accused of being codependent or "enablers" of infidelity; or, alternatively, they may be encouraged to "stand by your man" regardless of how unhealthy the relationship might be.

Working toward an informed decision about how best to respond to your partner's affair and whether to stay in the marriage—regardless of what decision you eventually reach—is neither foolish nor unhealthy. You shouldn't leave your marriage to avoid appearing weak any more than you should stay in your marriage to appear strong. How you appear to others isn't nearly as important as what's best for you in terms of your own long-term happiness and well-being. Be sure the decisions you reach are based on your own careful assessment of your partner, your marriage, and yourself—not on the values or biases of your extended family, your children, your friends, or, least of all, people with their own axes to grind and self-interests at heart.

How Am I Making This More Difficult for My Partner?

Your partner may also be struggling with thoughts and feelings about the affair, how it came about, and what's happened since. You can't resolve your partner's struggles, but you can avoid making your partner's recovery more difficult—not only for her sake but for your own sake and for the sake of the marriage.

Not Containing Your Emotions

As time goes on, it's important that you learn how to care for yourself, get a break from your intense negative feelings for both yourself and your partner, and find ways to calm yourself when your feelings threaten to get out of control. Repeatedly asking the same questions about the affair or having the same arguments, with the same intense feelings and without any progress, can eventually wear your partner out. That doesn't mean your partner doesn't have a responsibility to engage with you in discussions about how or why the affair happened, or what the implications are now; it does mean that both of you need an emotional break from continued turmoil. It also means that you're responsible for *how* you engage in these discussions with your partner.

When someone hurts you deeply, it's common to want to hurt him back—but deliberately punishing your partner needs to decrease and, it is hoped, comes to an end. That includes yelling at your partner for the affair or referring to the affair when others are around. It also includes withholding affection or other forms of positive interaction. We don't believe you should become physically or sexually intimate before you're emotionally ready—but when emotional or physical distance is used to punish or get even, such distancing behaviors become destructive to the marriage. Similarly, refusing to engage in warm or even casual discussions, rejecting genuine acts of caring from your partner, or avoiding opportunities for positive interactions of any kind may seem gratifying as an expression of anger in the short run while ending the marriage in the long run. You and your partner both need to have reasons to believe that the marriage can feel good again.

Undermining Your Partner's Relationships with Others

You and your partner will likely continue to have times when significant conflict or emotional distance comes between you. During these times it's important that your partner have *appropriate* sources of compassion and emotional support. You don't want your partner turning to the outside person as a significant source of caring and refuge while you struggle in your relationship. Consequently, it's important that you actively encourage and promote your partner's relationships with your children, extended family, or good friends who support your marriage. Speaking in harsh, critical ways about your partner to others who have been close and supportive to your partner in the past may provide some relief for you, but it does little to strengthen your marriage. Indeed, it may compromise those very relationships that provide the nurturing and compassion your partner needs to end the affair and refrain from any further interactions with the other person.

Failing to Reconcile Yourself to Uncertainty

Injured partners' need to understand the affair to the point where it "makes sense" usually stems from a belief that if they understood the partner's affair completely, they might be able to prevent it from happening again. But even after you two explore all the contributing factors to the best of your ability, the affair may never make sense to either of you. At some point, virtually everything that could contribute to understanding your partner's affair will have been discussed and there will be nothing new to add. Beyond that point of diminishing returns, continued "rehashing" of the same material is unproductive. It doesn't help you feel more secure, and it erodes any hope that your partner may have that the two of you can ever get beyond the affair.

249

Can you resign yourself to never completely understanding how your partner came to participate in an affair? At least to some extent, a decision to have an affair involves a degree of irrationality and emotional response that can never make complete sense. Can you move on to rebuild trust and intimacy with your partner knowing that you can never be absolutely certain that another affair couldn't happen? What are the potential costs to you and to your marriage if you can't find a way to do that?

Can I Keep an Affair from Happening Again?

If your partner becomes determined to have another affair, there's really nothing you can do to prevent it. You *may* be able to reduce the likelihood that your partner will have another affair. You can't change your partner's basic character and values, but you can challenge your partner to deal with aspects of herself that left her at greater risk for engaging in an affair. You can't single-handedly resolve all the difficulties in your marriage that made it more vulnerable to an affair, but you quite possibly can change your own contributions to conflict, emotional or physical distance, or susceptibility to outside stressors that increased the risk of an affair. Finally, you can examine any aspects of yourself that currently are making recovery for yourself or your partner more difficult and then work to change these for the sake of your marriage and your own well-being.

All of these efforts on your part will require a degree of trust. By definition, *trust* means not knowing for sure. You'll never know with complete certainty that your partner won't have another affair. The trust you need to have now if you decide to stay in your marriage is neither absolute nor blind. Rather, it's a measured trust that reflects your understanding of your partner and yourself, your relationship and the outside world, and whatever evidence you have of your partner's commitment to rebuild a relationship in which mutual caring, respect, and faithfulness guide partners' behaviors every day.

Reaching an informed decision about whether you and your partner can achieve this will require you to pull together all you've learned so far in Part II of this book. The next chapter will help you to do this.

Brenda, described at the beginning of this chapter, at first found it difficult to consider her own role in the marriage before Matt's affair. Most of her thoughts centered on how hard she had been trying to hold their marriage together and how misunderstood by Matt she had felt. However, as she gradually gained better control of her own feelings and her intense anger at Matt waned, she began to notice his efforts to be more involved at home—preparing dinner, managing bills, or proposing how to finance the home remodeling they had discussed. He didn't ask Brenda to excuse his previous behavior, and he seemed more willing to give her space when she struggled with flashbacks to his affair.

Matt ended his affair within a week after Brenda learned of it, and he drafted a letter to his former girlfriend affirming his decision, which he shared with Brenda before sending it. He stopped blaming Brenda for problems in their marriage, but also avoided talking with her about their marriage at all. At first Brenda felt relieved when Matt no longer pointed to her long hours at work as a reason for his affair, but his silence about his unhappiness in their marriage and Brenda's absences from home began to leave her feeling uneasy. Her relief that came from not talking about their marriage eventually turned into concern that they hadn't really fixed anything.

A turning point came one night when Brenda approached Matt and said she was still deeply hurt by his affair but was even more fearful that this could destroy their marriage if they didn't find a way to learn from it. She said there were things he needed to learn about himself but she was also willing to look at her own role in their marriage. She said she could see how Matt may have felt he wasn't as important to her as he had once been. After trying unsuccessfully to get Matt to talk with her about how he had viewed their marriage during his affair, Brenda finally exclaimed, "Look—at this point I'm less concerned about assigning blame than I am with getting this right. We just can't go on this way—with me worrying that you're too unhappy to stay, and you worrying that I'm too hurt or angry to look at what was going on in our marriage and how I was a part of it. Maybe we won't be able to make the marriage work in a way that feels right for both of us. But we won't even have a chance unless we're both willing to talk and listen. I need you to trust that I'm ready to do both."

More discussions were necessary before Brenda and Matt came to a fuller understanding of how their marriage had become vulnerable and what each of them would need to do now to deal with the chal-

251

lenges in and outside their home without losing the emotional connection that had held them together previously through difficult times. Brenda's willingness to look at her own contributions to their marriage provided Matt with courage to do the same on his part. Their recovery wasn't easy. The challenges of balancing the needs of their relationship with the pressures of their respective careers at times seemed overwhelming. But struggling with these challenges together began to produce greater understanding and closeness, in contrast to the distance they had both felt previously.

What's Next?

If you're the injured partner, complete the following exercises to help you take a closer look at your role in making the marriage more vulnerable to an affair and making recovery more difficult—either for yourself or your partner—than it needs to be. If you're the participating partner, and the injured partner isn't yet ready to do these exercises, keep your own responses available and, following our earlier advice on page 235, express your willingness to discuss these issues later when your partner feels more willing and able. In the next chapter we'll help you both review the work you've done in the last four chapters, pull out the most important insights you've gained, and use these to construct a more coherent, integrated "narrative" or story of how the affair occurred.

———————— Exercises ————————

EXERCISE 10.1. ASPECTS OF THE INJURED PARTNER CONTRIBUTING TO VULNERABILITY TO AN AFFAIR

To get the clearest understanding of what happened that made your marriage vulnerable to an affair, it's important to understand the injured partner's role in the relationship and the affair. We encourage you to do this in two ways. First, are there ways that the injured partner wasn't meeting the needs of the person who had the affair? Not meeting someone's needs doesn't justify an affair, but examining this question can promote an understanding of the setting in which the person responded by having an affair. Second, while the affair was developing or ongoing, were there aspects of the injured partner that made it hard to recognize or respond to the affair or made it more difficult to end it?

Look back at your relationship prior to the affair. Make a list of ways that the injured partner (1) wasn't meeting the needs of the person who had the affair or (2) wasn't doing his or her part to make the relationship work. For example:

"I have to admit that as I got busier at work, when I came home I wasn't fully present. I was so caught up in dealing with my own issues that I didn't take time to hear about his day. Although he shouldn't have had the affair, I guess he found someone who wanted to listen."

Or

"I'm just not the romantic type; she's really much more that way than I am. I have to accept major responsibility for letting the romance die in our relationship. I know she wanted more than sex; she wanted us to have romance, and I didn't do my part."

Look back to the time when the relationship with the outside person was developing or the affair was taking place. Clarify and write down the factors that may have made it hard for the injured partner to recognize that an inappropriate relationship was developing or more difficult to demand that the affair come to an end. For example, as the injured partner, you might now realize:

"I've never been able to stand up for myself when I talk with my husband. I was afraid that if I confronted him with my suspicions about his affair, somehow I'd look stupid or he wouldn't even respond—so I just kept quiet for much too long."

Or, as the participating partner:

"I think he loved me so much and had such dreams for our marriage that he just couldn't allow himself to see that my 'friendship' with the other man wasn't just a friendship. His wish to keep the dream alive made him deny what was happening, and then we just couldn't talk about it."

EXERCISE 10.2. ASPECTS OF THE INJURED PARTNER
THAT HELP OR HINDER RECOVERY

When either of you examine the role of the injured partner, you may discover some things that make it difficult for that person to recover from the affair or make it hard for the participating partner to recover. Likewise, perhaps the injured partner has qualities or is behaving in ways that will help the recovery.

Make two lists. First, list things that the injured partner is doing or aspects of that person that make it more difficult for either person to recover from the affair. For example:

> "Although I hate to admit it, anytime someone hurts me, I want to get that person back. I don't typically move on until I've had my revenge. I know she's sorry and will probably never do it again, but I can't seem to help it. I continue to attack her over and over, even though I can see it's driving another wedge between us."

> Or

> "I still can't stand up to him to say what I need to say or ask the questions I need to ask. There's so much we really need to understand if we're going to get beyond this, but I can't get myself to bring it up. If I don't find a way to discuss the affair in more detail, I'm afraid I may stay silent and miserable forever."

Second, list strengths or positive qualities that the injured partner has that might help in recovery from the affair. For example:

> "Even when I've been hurt badly by someone, if I see that we can make things work, I'm able to forgive and do whatever work is needed to repair things. I try to learn from the past, not live in it."

11

How Do I Make Sense
of It All?

"Making sense of it all" is less about "why" the affair occurred and more about "how" it happened. How did the marriage become vulnerable? What went wrong? What failed to go right? What would have to happen now to restore confidence and security in your marriage? If you've worked through Chapters 7 to 10, you've already accomplished much of the work to answer these questions. Nevertheless, given the sheer volume of everything you've considered—as well as the distress you've likely struggled with along the way—it may have been difficult to pull all the pieces together in a way that allows you to see the big picture. This chapter is intended to help you with this challenge. We'll guide you through the process of reviewing the work you've already done, pulling out the most important insights you've gained, and using these to construct a coherent narrative or accounting of the affair.

How Do I Sort Through Everything
I've Learned?

The first step is to review the work you completed in previous chapters. If you haven't yet completed the exercises for the preceding four chapters, it's important that you work through those now. Exploring the full range of influences that could have contributed to this affair is critical to identifying what's most important and understanding how these influences interacted with each other.

Ideally, you and your partner have each worked through these exercises and have already discussed your responses. If not, it's still not too late to encourage your partner to join you in this effort. If working through the previous chapters separately has been helpful to you in interacting with your partner more positively, discuss these changes with your partner and describe how things could be even better if your partner would join you in the process. If he or she hasn't already done so, ask your partner to read Chapter 6—if nothing else—to understand why engaging in this process together is so important to you. If your partner hasn't pursued this with you but agrees to try it now, be patient as your partner works to catch up with you. Go slowly, taking one chapter at a time, discussing your perspectives and trying to build some common ground before going on to the next one.

Then—whether separately or with your partner—review your responses to each of the exercises. From everything you've learned, now try to highlight the most important contributing factors you've identified. Sometimes people overlook important factors when first working through a chapter but recognize such factors more clearly after working through subsequent chapters. An important part of this process is to determine the specific role that any contributing factor played in *your* marriage. For example, if you identify "relationships with in-laws" as a stressor in the marriage that caused tensions between you and your partner, pinpoint what the specific conflicts with your in-laws involved, what negative effects they had on interactions between you and your partner, and what steps would be involved in reducing these difficulties.

After you've reviewed your responses to each of the preceding four chapters and have highlighted the most important contributing factors that you've identified, try to sort these into the following three categories:

- Negative influences and stressors that placed your marriage at risk (for example, high levels of conflict or feeling emotionally or physically disconnected).
- Positive qualities that contributed to increased risk (for example, leadership skills resulting in too many outside commitments).
- Absence of adequate protective factors (for example, lack of involvement in social groups or activities that support your marriage).

Then, within each of these categories, divide these factors into two groups based on when they were most important: (1) before the affair or (2) during or after the affair. A little later in this chapter, we'll show you how one couple introduced earlier—Nick and Becky—completed a worksheet to pull together their understanding of what happened in their own marriage.

How do you determine what's most important? There's no simple answer to this essential question. What appears insignificant to one partner can seem vitally important to the other. Conflicts with the children may have occurred more frequently or had greater impact for one parent than the other, or one partner may have felt more stressed by financial concerns than the other. You may differ in how much threat you perceive from outside your marriage or how protective you believe relationships with others who support your marriage are. It's not essential that you and your partner agree completely on every factor you identify as contributing to vulnerability to an affair. It *is* important that there be substantial overlap in your perspectives and that each of you acknowledge and tolerate the other's viewpoint.

How Do I Pull the Pieces Together into a Coherent Picture?

Developing a coherent picture of the affair is like filming a movie with a wide-angle lens. You need the wide-angle lens to make sure everything that's relevant shows up on the screen; a too narrow lens leaves out some important details entirely and leaves other details out of focus and distorted. You also need a wide-angle lens to see how the different characters and forces interact and influence each other. Watching a character jump off a bridge may not make sense until you see the wider view that shows a car careening wildly toward that person after one of the tires blows out.

Similarly, a meaningful understanding of the affair is more like a movie than a photograph. You need to know how things developed over time, not just at one particular point such as when the affair began.

In short, the narrative or story you develop for the affair needs to have a beginning, a middle, and—we hope—an end.

In Chapter 9, you met Nick and Becky and read about Nick's affair with a business associate, Diana. After reviewing their efforts to identify contributing factors to the affair from within and outside their marriage, as well as in themselves, Nick and Becky completed the worksheet shown on the next page. Later each of them used this worksheet to prepare a written narrative that expressed their best understanding of how Nick's affair had come about—a process we'll describe later in this chapter.

In evaluating the various factors that contributed to your relationship being at risk for an affair, be sure to include:

- What was going on in your marriage and with each of you before an affair was even considered.
- What experiences you and your partner had growing up in your families that influenced your behaviors with each other and in regard to the affair.
- What happened that actually triggered the affair.
- What possibly contributed to the affair's continuing.
- What has made it more difficult for you or your partner to recover.

Nick and Becky recognized that they had gradually allowed themselves to drift apart while devoting nearly all their time and energy to work and their children. This had interfered first with their feeling close emotionally and then with their physical intimacy. They also had given up some of their important friendships with people who had helped their marriage through difficult times in the past. Although Nick and Becky rarely had major arguments, their reluctance to address ongoing concerns in their marriage led to a steady undercurrent of tension and irritability. Their sexual relationship seemed particularly difficult to discuss. Nick didn't want to pressure Becky, so he generally avoided physical contact that suggested any interest in sex; Becky interpreted his physical withdrawal as a lack of attraction to her, which felt hurtful and caused her to be reluctant to initiate sex or other physical closeness.

Both Nick and Becky recognized that other people found Nick easy to interact with and that women often found him to be more sensitive and understanding than most of the men they knew. But they also now recognized that Nick's warm and easy way of interacting with women could trigger feelings of attraction that also required clear boundaries, which Nick had sometimes been reluctant to set. The marriage had entered a crisis before either one of them fully recognized what was happening.

After ending his affair, Nick had begged for Becky's understanding but couldn't yet bring himself to ask for her forgiveness. In fact, the depth

Sample Worksheet Completed by Nick and Becky

	Factors having an influence before the affair	Factors having an influence during and following the affair
Negative influences and stressors (your marriage, outside factors, your partner, you)	Frequent irritability and "nitpicking" Differences in needs for spontaneity vs. predictability Low levels of physical intimacy Intrusions into relationship time from work and children Admiration and pursuit by another, combined with Nick's enduring self-doubts Nick's inattention to risks and need for boundaries	Becky's discomfort with talking about sex Nick's capacity for compartmentalizing or separating things mentally Becky's withdrawal in response to hurt or disappointment Nick's feelings of shame that blocked discussions of the affair
Positive qualities contributing to risk (your marriage, outside factors, your partner, you)	Nick's physical attractiveness and personal warmth Both partners' strong work ethic Both partners' devotion to their children	Becky's tolerance for emotional distance based on her confidence that things would eventually improve on their own Nick's reluctance to express unhappiness in their marriage Nick's emotional attachment to Diana
Absence of protective factors that reduce the risk of an affair	Failure to set apart time for the marriage as a couple	Both partners' retreat from supportive relationships

of Nick's guilt and shame had initially made it difficult for him to even talk with Becky about his affair after he had ended it. The depth of Becky's hurt and her tendency to retreat when feeling wounded, along with the depth of Nick's shame, which became even greater when he recognized the pain he had caused Becky, were barriers to working together that required considerable effort to overcome, just to begin a process toward recovery. Only because of their genuine caring for each other and a commitment to preserving their family, if possible, were Nick and Becky able to survive the initial impact of Nick's affair and gradually work toward the understanding reflected in the worksheet they prepared together.

After completing this worksheet, Nick and Becky each prepared a written narrative that expressed their best understanding of how Nick's affair had come about. Both wrote their narratives in the form of a letter—something they had learned to do as a way of communicating initially about difficult issues when working through Chapter 3 and struggling with the initial impact of the affair.

What Does a Narrative of the Affair Look Like?

Following is Becky's initial narrative of Nick's affair—a good example of efforts to develop a picture that's both complete and balanced.

Dear Nick,

I've worked so hard to make sense of your affair. I know you've worked hard too, and I want you to know how important that has been to me. I don't think I could have done this on my own. I needed your support and your help. I had to know that you needed to understand this as much as I do, and that you were willing to struggle through this with me.

Your affair will never make complete sense to me. There were so many choice points along the way—I wish we could both go back and do things differently. We could have avoided so much terrible heartache for us both. The best we can do now is to try to learn from what's happened. I need to know that we've both learned from this, Nick—that we each understand as best we can how we ended up here, what we each contributed to this situation, and what we're committed to doing differently. I need to know that, as much as possible, we're each doing everything we can to make sure that nothing like this ever happens again. I don't think I could survive that, Nick, and I actually don't think that you could either.

We took each other and our marriage for granted. That's hard to admit, but I know that at some level it's true. We let our work and our children get in the way; we didn't protect our own relationship. I guess I was so certain of you and certain of us that I never even imagined that our marriage could get in trouble. We each put the children first in ways that ended up harming us and potentially harming them, too, if we don't find a way to move beyond what's happened. We both let work take priority, when we should have been protecting us for the sake of our family.

I know we had our differences, Nick, but none of them ever seemed that big to me. You've said that you thought I was often irritable and gave you the cold shoulder, and that you didn't think I liked you very much anymore. I didn't mean to be irritable. I think I was just always feeling under pressure to keep everything perfect and not disappoint you. Sometimes when I withdrew from you I was just trying to give you time and space for yourself. I didn't understand that you thought I just didn't need you as much anymore.

I understand now that my efforts to keep things perfect had more to do with me than with your needs. You've always been more comfortable with just acting on the moment, when I've preferred things to be orderly and predictable. For me, structure was how I kept our family from becoming chaotic like my own family when I was growing up. For me, routines felt safe and secure. For you, they felt controlling and restricting—and I guess I reminded you of the way your mom was with you. We've done better lately in finding a healthier balance. Sometimes I just remind myself to loosen up, and I've seen how sometimes you understand and support my need for routines—especially with the kids.

You and I never really argued and I guess that made me feel secure because we didn't have the kinds of awful fights that my parents used to have. I know we nitpicked, but I never let it get to me too much; I just tried to go about my business and wait for the tension to pass. I could see the pained look on your face sometimes, but you never said very much. We just went to our separate corners. We need to keep working on handling those times better, Nick. We each need to be more mindful about our irritability. But more important, I really want you to come to me and let me know when you're feeling hurt or upset. And I'll try to do a better job of seeking you out when I see that you've pulled back. I see you as so "strong" that I forget that you're also tender. I do love your tenderness, Nick; it's one of the reasons I was attracted to you.

I'll try to reach out to you when I'm feeling hurt, too. I know I tend to pull back into my shell. It's how I survive, something I learned growing up. I'll work harder at letting you know when I'm hurt or disappointed, but I need for you to be able to hear me without feeling like I'm condemning you as some terrible person. You and I both work so hard to be good people that it's hard for us to admit when we've made mistakes or fallen short. I understand better now that this kind of defensiveness gets in the way of positive change. I know we've both been working on this, but I think we'll have to get even better if we're going to protect our marriage and keep it on track.

Nick, I know it's hard for me to talk with you about our physical relationship—about sex. It's even hard for me to write that word. I don't understand completely why that is, but I know it's been a problem for us. Between the stresses of work and the children, combined with wanting everything at home in order and chores done before being able to relax, I just wasn't in the mood for lovemaking as often as you were. And then you started to pull back from me and didn't hold me or kiss me as often, and gradually we just became more and more physically distant. Even holding hands or sitting close together on the couch fell by the wayside. Nick, I do like our lovemaking. I do crave being touched and held by you. I don't believe you ever understood how much I missed our physical closeness, too. You just thought I didn't need or desire you, so you pulled back, and that made me feel even worse and made me think that maybe you didn't desire me anymore. I know I don't have the same figure I had when we married and I worry about that, even though you tell me not to.

When you told me about your affair with Diana I just completely fell apart. It confirmed all my worst fears—that I couldn't compete with other women who were younger, prettier, or more successful and a part of the world where you work. I wasn't just hurt, Nick. I was devastated. And completely panicked because I didn't see any way that I could compete— and, to be honest, I wasn't sure I wanted to. Once I realized that you had feelings for her—and it wasn't just about sex—that made it even worse. I couldn't understand why you found it hard just to cut her out of your life. I was so incredibly hurt and frightened that I couldn't even look at you because it made the pain worse. Did that make it harder for you to end it with her, when I shut down, because you were afraid of ending up completely alone?

I don't want us to stay married because of the kids, Nick. I only want us to stay married if we can devote ourselves to each other in all the right ways. I don't think we can do this all on our own. Before your affair we became really isolated from our friends. We stopped going out with other couples. The only other people we spent time with were our families, and those times weren't always particularly enjoyable—especially on my side. I want us to start going out with other couples again, like we did before the kids were born. And I want us both to take time to renew the separate friendships that were good for us. After you told me about your affair, I drew back from my friends because I was just too embarrassed—in part about you, but also about me. I just felt so inadequate. And I know you cut off some of your friends, too, because you felt like a "fraud" as you say. But we have to get back to having good friendships because I think these help us be better in our own friendship.

Nick, you know I'll never excuse your affair, and I now believe that you never will either. Nothing will ever make that affair "right." But we can try to learn from the past to make the present and our future better. I think we've been making progress, but I don't want to stop working together. There are things we each still need to work on.

I do love you, Nick. That's why this work is so important to me.

Becky

Nick's narrative was briefer. Although he understood and agreed with the contributing factors he and Becky had identified, he still shied away from emphasizing these—mostly because he continued to struggle with remorse and preferred to focus on his own role. However, Becky had asked him to work with her toward the "bigger picture," and he tried to do so.

Dear Becky,

After all this time, I still hardly know where to begin. What I want to say most is how very sorry I am. Those words seem so empty. I don't know how to express how horrible I feel every time I think about what I did to you—and to us. I know that my feeling guilty won't make things right again—you've told me before that I need to get unstuck from my guilt to focus on what needs to change. I hope you can see by now that I'm committed to doing whatever it takes to make our marriage work. But I also want you to know that however good we're able to make it—I'll never forget how I almost threw it away.

I also want you to know how grateful I am that you've hung in there. Even when you were feeling the most hurt by me—so hurt you could hardly speak to me—I don't think you ever completely gave up on us. I don't know if I could have been as strong as you've been if the situation were reversed. Your strength through this terrible ordeal is another reminder to me of how incredibly special you are and how lucky I am to have you in my life.

Looking back, I still don't understand how I did what I did. I understand that things weren't going all that well between us at home, and that we each had a lot going on in our lives. And I understand better how maybe I never really came to grips with how I think about myself before now—how I've probably wrestled with those "demons" of inadequacy for a long time. But I want you to know that—putting that all together—it still doesn't add up to what I let myself get involved in. I need you to know that no matter how bad it ever gets in the future—even if a thousand times worse—I'll never again let myself cave in to self-pity to look for reassurance elsewhere. If nothing else, this whole situation has forced me to take a hard look at myself and grow up in ways I just didn't see before.

Becky, maybe we both took our marriage for granted, but I probably did the most. I let my role as "breadwinner" justify abandoning you with most of the responsibilities at home, and then when you weren't there for me at times or in ways that I wanted, I felt sorry for myself. When I couldn't get you to spend time with me, I'd go off with my friends, and that seemed to annoy you even more. We've already talked some about how to change this. I feel good about leaving work earlier to be home for dinner and evenings with you and the kids. And I can tell the difference it's made for you, too, when I'm around more. You seem less hassled—more relaxed with yourself and less irritated with me.

I'm sorry you thought I lost interest in you—that I didn't want to make love with you anymore. Becky, I've always thought you were beautiful, and I loved what we did in bed together. It wasn't just about the sex—although that was great, too. It's the way you held on to me so tight during and after sex, and the way we could then fall asleep together or get up an hour later like all the tensions between us had just melted away. I felt closer to you when we made love—it was the feeling between us afterward that meant the most to me. When we didn't have sex, and then we didn't have that feeling afterward, that's when I started to feel the most alone. I know I *should have done a better job of explaining that, and I also should have done better at finding out what it took for you to feel closer to me. I think we've been doing a lot better in the past couple of months—balancing the different ways we get close together—not just sex, but other ways, too.*

Becky, I admire how responsible you are. You're an incredible mom for our kids. You make our home a good place to live. I appreciate all you do to keep things in order and to plan special events for us. Sometimes, though, I enjoy it the most when you just laugh and get silly with me and the kids, and when things aren't so planned and we can just be who we are with each other. I understand better now why predictability is important to you—and how scary it must have been for you growing up when you could never predict who was going to be home when, or what kind of mood your dad was going to be in, or whether your mom was going to be too depressed to get herself dressed or get meals on the table. I think we've been getting better about this, too. Our kids don't need as much "hands on" care anymore, and I actually enjoy working with them after dinner to get the kitchen cleaned up so you can have time for yourself before you and I get back together. Going for walks by ourselves or just getting out of the house together for half an hour without worrying so much about chores or what the kids are doing has been a really nice change.

You've said we should go out with other couples more, and I agree. Becky, I just felt like such a huge hypocrite that I couldn't bear being around other couples who seemed to get along so well when I could only think of how I had betrayed you, the kids, and the most important promise of my life I made on our wedding day. We need to surround ourselves with other people who can support us and our marriage. It's been too easy to feel like the "lone ranger" out there—all alone—and I clearly got lost along the way.

Becky, I adore you. You've been the most wonderful and precious gift of my life. I will never, ever lose sight of that again, and—if you'll still have me—I promise I will do whatever it takes to keep you and our marriage as the focus of my life forever.

Love,

Nick

After Becky and Nick had each written their own narratives of Nick's affair, they exchanged and read them in private. They took a few days to reflect on what they had each written and identify where they saw things similarly and where they differed. For example, although Nick acknowledged being frustrated with the lack of sex before his affair, he emphasized that this hadn't been nearly as important as feeling emotionally distant from Becky and their lack of playtime together. Similarly, Becky clarified that Nick's time with his male friends hadn't troubled her nearly as much as Nick had believed and that, in fact, she sensed that Nick was sometimes invigorated and more enthusiastic about family life after a day off with his friends.

Following this discussion, Becky and Nick each revised their narratives and again exchanged and discussed them. Their revisions not only included some of the corrected understandings that had come from their previous discussion, but also emphasized some of the steps they had already taken to make things better over the prior months and how those efforts had helped.

How Do I Share This Work with My Partner?

Despite your best efforts, your partner still may not be ready or willing to join you in this process. If so, we again encourage you to consider the suggestions provided in Chapter 6 for each of you working separately, or for you by yourself, in making sense of the affair. For example, your partner may be willing to review the worksheet of contributing factors that you've constructed (Exercise 11.1) or to read through your narrative (Exercise 11.2) and then discuss his or her reactions. If your partner won't participate even at this level, it's important that you go ahead and do this work by yourself anyway. Your partner may eventually recognize the importance of this work and accept the challenge of exploring the context for the affair. Even if your partner doesn't take part in this process, you'll have a better understanding of how the affair came about and reach better decisions about how to move forward—whether in the marriage or separately on your own—if you go through this exploration process and then complete the worksheet and construct a narrative of the affair as we've described here.

What's Next?

Complete the following exercises, first using the worksheet to summarize your understanding of the factors that contributed to the affair and then writing a narrative or story of the affair, using everything you've learned to pull together a more complete picture. Take your time in working through these exercises. *They may be some of the most important work you'll do to recover from the affair.*

Then go on to the last part of this book, which focuses on decisions about how to move forward. In Chapter 12, we'll help you examine ways of moving beyond the hurt feelings and the negative thoughts or behaviors that may at times still keep you tied to the past rather than working toward your future. Chapter 13 will guide you toward decisions about whether to stay in your marriage or move on separately—and how best to implement whichever decision you reach. Finally, Chapter 14 examines additional challenges that lie ahead and how to stay focused on a healthier future.

Exercises

EXERCISE 11.1. CONSTRUCTING A SUMMARY OF IMPORTANT FACTORS CONTRIBUTING TO THE AFFAIR

As you've worked through the last few chapters, you've already developed a better understanding of what contributed to the affair. This set of exercises will help you pull together everything you've learned into one coherent picture. *In this first exercise, fill in a copy of the worksheet on page 269, summarizing what you see as the important factors contributing to the affair, or construct your own version of the same form.* Look back at your responses to the exercises for Chapters 7 through 10, which can serve as the basis for this summary. Try to include important aspects of both your relationship and influences outside your relationship, as well as aspects of both your partner and yourself.

Throughout this process, try to include not only negative factors, but also positive aspects of your relationship or of you and your partner that may have been important factors. For example, if you have extensive commitments to your extended family or to groups in the community, these can leave little time for your relationship. In addition, successful careers can be stressful as well as helping you feel better about yourself. Try to keep your summary of contributing factors balanced, focused, and not overwhelming. For example, try not to leave any cell in the worksheet entirely blank, and try to limit yourself to five or six items in any particular category.

EXERCISE 11.2.
PREPARING AND EXCHANGING A NARRATIVE OF THE AFFAIR

In your own words, write a narrative or story of what you see as the major factors that contributed to the affair or created the context for it. Use the worksheet you just created to develop your story of how the affair came about. Remember to include any long-standing risk factors, more recent influences that may have triggered the affair or contributed to its continuing, and factors that have made it more difficult for you or your partner to recover. *In short, make sure your story of the affair has a beginning, a middle, and an end.* Some people write better than others; don't worry about your writing skills or how long your story is. What's most important is the understanding that you convey in your narrative and how well the story fits together and explains the affair for you and your partner—not how great a writer you are.

If your partner hasn't been reading the book or hasn't been doing the exercises, then still write out your own story. If your partner is willing to read it, give it to your partner when you've finished; we hope that will lead to a useful discussion. If your partner isn't willing to read your narrative, write it anyway. It will give you greater understanding, and perhaps your partner will be more willing to read it in the future.

After preparing your narratives, you and your partner should exchange and discuss them, using specific steps for doing this:

1. Exchange and read each other's narrative or story separately.
2. Discuss with your partner how you saw things similarly and differently.
3. If this discussion gives you new insights, revise your narrative, but don't feel you have to see things exactly as your partner does.
4. Exchange and discuss these revisions.
5. Acknowledge any remaining differences in understanding between the two of you.
6. Focus on what you see in common and how you can use that to move forward in the future.

Worksheet for Summarizing Factors Related to the Affair

	Factors having an influence before the affair	Factors having an influence during and following the affair
Negative influences and stressors (your marriage, outside factors, your partner, you)		
Positive qualities contributing to risk (your marriage, outside factors, your partner, you)		
Absence of protective factors that reduce the risk of an affair		

From *Getting Past the Affair* by Douglas K. Snyder, Donald H. Baucon, and Kristina Coop Gordon. Copyright 2007 by The Guilford Press.

>>>

Part III

CAN THIS MARRIAGE BE SAVED?

12

How Do I Get Past the Hurt?

"I'm still having trouble getting past it," Wendy said softly. "Ross has done everything I've asked and more. For the most part, we're doing a lot better now than we were six months ago. But sometimes when I think about his affair, I still get angry and lash out at him. I say ugly things I don't even really mean, and then afterward I usually feel even worse. Most of the time, Ross just takes it or walks off without saying anything. But I know he feels beaten down when I lash out like that. Last week he asked me whether I'd ever get over it. What's that supposed to mean? Am I supposed to forget it ever happened? I can't just forget it—even though sometimes I wish I could. I don't think I want Ross to forget it either. Maybe remembering all the pain we've been through since his affair will help keep him from ever doing something like that again. I just wish I knew what to do with the resentment I still feel and how to move on."

Even after you've worked to understand how your partner's affair came about and addressed factors that put your marriage at risk, hurt feelings can linger. When there's little relief from the hurt and the painful feelings remain too strong or resurface too frequently, they not only get in the way of emotional closeness but eventually do even more damage to you and your relationship. Finding a way to move past the deep hurt of your partner's affair is a crucial part of recovery.

Chronic, unresolved hurt and the anger that frequently accompanies that hurt are simply unhealthy, emotionally and physically. Considerable research shows that long-lasting hurt and anger frequently lead to depression, difficulties with sleep or with appetite (eating either too little or too much), decreases in sexual desire, irritability toward friends or coworkers, high blood pressure, muscle tension, headaches or back pain, and both emotional and physical fatigue. To counteract these effects, some people turn to alcohol or increase their reliance on medications.

The more successful you've been in working through the previous chapters, the more likely you've already made good progress in working past your hurt. But everyone is different. Some people continue to feel deep hurt that interferes with their day-to-day lives both in and outside their relationship even after working through the first two stages of recovery. Others, like Wendy, wrestle with feeling hurt and having memories of the affair at least occasionally.

What does it take, then, to move past the hurt once and for all? In this chapter we'll help you consider what "moving on" or "letting go" might mean and how doing so relates to beliefs you already have about forgiveness. We'll help you identify steps you or your partner can take toward moving past the hurt, as well as some of the barriers that may be making this more difficult. As you work through this chapter, however, try to remember that *feelings are usually harder to change than behaviors.* It's easier to choose how to act—and even choose how to think—than to choose how to feel. Because it's so hard to change your feelings, it's going to take time, even when you and your partner are doing everything "right." So try to be patient and encouraging to each other.

What Does It Mean to "Move On"?

Like Wendy, you may be struggling with questions about what it means to "move on." Does it mean never thinking of the affair again, or never feeling hurt or angry about it? Does it mean no longer holding your partner (or yourself) accountable? When people talk about moving on, they often mean different things—in terms of what it would look like at the end or what it would take to get there. We begin with describing what moving on looks like at the end, because knowing where you want to end up is important before constructing a road map that will lead you there.

>>> **Couples who move on after a deep personal injury like a partner's affair achieve four important goals:**
- **They regain a balanced view of the partner and their relationship.**
- **They commit not to let their hurt or anger rule their thoughts and behavior toward the partner or dominate their lives.**
- **They voluntarily give up the right to continue punishing the partner for his or her actions or demanding further restitution.**
- **They decide whether to continue in the relationship based on a realistic assessment of both its positive and negative qualities.**

Achieving a balanced view involves adopting a big-picture perspective that considers both positive and negative qualities. It requires viewing your partner not just in terms of the affair but also in light of everything else you've come to understand about your partner and your relationship. Making a commitment not to let your hurt or anger take over your life doesn't mean never hurting or feeling resentful again. It means working at not allowing those feelings to consume you. It requires recognizing when negative feelings about the affair resurface and then choosing to respond in ways that will be more constructive than simply lashing out. It involves redirecting your thoughts and actions toward current or future goals, rather than being overwhelmed by past hurt.

For some people, having the person who hurt you make amends can be an important part of moving on. Although nothing can undo an affair, acts of restitution or going "above and beyond" to show caring, concern, and love can sometimes serve as concrete expressions of remorse or a commitment to change. But demanding restitution—or punishing the participating partner—beyond a certain point doesn't strengthen the marriage or promote feelings of closeness. Continued vengeance may feel satisfying in the short run, but it almost always keeps you firmly stuck in the past in the long run.

When people choose to stay in a relationship, moving on means committing to a process of strengthening and maintaining the relationship, even during difficult times. You haven't moved on if you stay in the relationship but with one foot out the door. Uncertainty that's allowed to drag on that way saps the very energy necessary to make the relationship work. If, however, you choose to leave the relationship, moving on separately means no longer dwelling on the affair or your partner. It means redirecting your thoughts and behaviors toward building a new life.

Moving On: Possibly Forgiving but Not Necessarily Forgetting?

Moving on, letting go, and *forgiving* are terms that people often use interchangeably. Everyone has beliefs about what it means to forgive—although often these beliefs are hard to put into words. Sometimes these beliefs come from experiences of being forgiven (or not forgiven) in the past. Maybe you have clear memories of how your parents dealt with being hurt in their own relationship or how they dealt with you when you did something that disappointed or hurt them. Or your thoughts and feelings about forgiving may be more strongly influenced by how you and your partner have dealt with hurt between you in the past. Can you remember times when you and your partner disappointed or hurt each other, but the two of you found a way to put those feelings behind you and either moved on or "started fresh"? Can you remember times when either one of you was unable to get past hurt feelings and what impact that had on your relationship?

People's beliefs about forgiveness are also often closely linked to their religious beliefs. In some religious traditions, people are forgiven only after they've confessed to wrongdoing and expressed remorse, as well as compensated the hurt person in some way and vowed to avoid the situations that caused the hurt. In other traditions, forgiveness may be offered to someone regardless of whether the person is remorseful or takes responsibility for the hurtful behavior. From this perspective, a decision by the injured person to forgive or "let go" involves giving up resentment and viewing the wrongdoer with compassion, even though the offending person may not be asking for forgiveness. What would forgiving your partner mean to you? Is forgiveness something you're willing to offer?

It's important to understand exactly what *you* mean by forgiveness so that you know what you can live with and in what ways you truly want to move on. Does forgiving mean pardoning to you? Pardoning someone for an offense generally releases him from further punishment or restitution—without necessarily having any implications for how you feel about the person. In most religious traditions, forgiving goes beyond pardoning: When you forgive someone, you also experience some "softening of the heart" toward him. To reconcile with someone, in contrast, means to restore a healed relationship. Although it's probably impossible to reconcile without first forgiving, people can forgive without reconciling. For example, you could say to someone, "I no longer want to punish you. I understand what led you to do what you did. I can see your remorse, and I'm sorry for your own suffering. However, I don't believe this relationship can be a healthy one for me, and I need to end it."

There's no doubt that forgiveness is a profound concept, so it's no wonder that it's often misunderstood. *Some common beliefs about forgiveness can interfere with moving on:*

- I need to forgive someone who apologizes, whether I want to or not.
- Forgiving someone means excusing what she did or saying that what happened is okay.
- Forgiving someone for hurtful or wrong actions requires compromising my own values about what's right.
- Some behaviors (for example, affairs or violence) shouldn't be forgiven.
- Forgiveness can't occur until compensation or restitution has been made.
- To forgive someone means no longer thinking about what he did.
- Forgiving someone means no longer feeling hurt or angry about what happened.
- Forgiving someone means leaving myself open to being hurt again.
- If I forgive someone, I need to stay in a relationship with that person.

Have you held beliefs similar to any of these? Which ones stand out for you? Would you add any? Try looking at these beliefs in light of what we've discussed so far. How might any of these beliefs be helpful to you in moving past your own hurt feelings—and how might they get in the way?

Let us make our own views on the meaning of forgiveness very clear:

- *Forgiving your partner **doesn't** mean approving of what she's done.* No matter how understanding you may be about what contributed to your partner's affair, you're unlikely ever to believe that it was the "right" choice or a good one.

 • *Similarly, forgiving your partner **isn't** the same as excusing or justifying what he's done.* You and your partner may have worked hard to understand how the affair came about or what factors put your relationship at risk. But contributing factors aren't excuses, just as explanations aren't justifications.

 • *Finally, forgiving your partner **doesn't** mean forgetting about the offense or no longer hurting from it.* You and your partner will continue to have times when you think about the affair, and those times may be accompanied by feelings of hurt, resentment, guilt, anxiety, or sadness. But moving on means working to minimize those thoughts and feelings by focusing on opportunities for pursuing a happy and productive life in the present and in the future. By itself, the passage of time helps but rarely heals deep emotional wounds. Moving on, letting go, and forgiving all require commitment to a process that will help you reach this goal and actively taking steps to move forward.

What Are the Steps to Moving On?

There's no single sequence of events or universal time line that works well for everyone. The specific steps may vary, depending on the factors contributing to the affair, your beliefs about forgiveness, your partner's behaviors, and consequences of the affair for you or for others—such as your children. The steps we'll describe over the next few pages represent a process that fits for many people. Not all of these steps may be relevant or essential for your own moving on, and the order of these steps may be different for you. Use the following discussion and Exercise 12.1 to think about what events seem important to *you* for moving on. Which of these have you and your partner already achieved? Which ones still lie before you— and how could you help to bring these about?

Recognition

Step 1 involves the offending partner's developing a clear understanding of what happened and its consequences. Think back to the material in Chapter 3 about discussing your feelings about the affair. Did you and your partner exchange letters as suggested in the exercises for that chapter? If not, were you able to have a thorough and helpful discussion about the impact of the affair? If you didn't complete the exercises for that chapter or if important aspects of understanding the impact of the affair still seem not to be recognized or understood, reread that chapter or ask your partner to read and discuss the chapter with you.

Steps to Moving On Past Hurt and Anger

- **Recognition**: The participating partner develops and expresses a clear understanding of the affair and its consequences.
- **Responsibility**: The participating partner takes full responsibility for decisions and choices related to the affair.
- **Remorse**: The participating partner expresses genuine feelings of deep sadness, mourning, or even pain from the hurt he or she has caused.
- **Restitution**: The participating partner engages in positive actions intended to minimize the hurt and related negative consequences stemming from his or her actions.
- **Reform**: The participating partner provides reassurance and evidence of a commitment not to hurt the injured partner in the future by:
  —Pledging not to hurt the injured partner in the same way again.
  —Addressing conditions that contributed to the previous affair.
  —Acting differently when confronted with similar situations in the future.
- **Release**: The injured partner commits to a process of "letting go" or moving on, voluntarily giving up the right to continue punishing his or her partner for the affair or demanding further restitution.
- **Reconciliation**: Both partners commit to rebuilding a relationship based on mutual trust and caring.

Responsibility

Affairs don't "just happen." They involve a decision—either explicit or implicit—to cross the line and engage in a behavior that almost always has been defined ahead of time by the couple as not acceptable. Couples can get stuck in the recovery process, and injured partners can find it particularly difficult to move past their hurt if the participating partner persists in declaring, "I never meant to hurt you." Although usually not intended as such, this statement conveys a continued failure to take responsibility for avoiding or actively resisting an affair. Injured partners frequently can't move on until the person who had the affair takes responsibility for his choices throughout the affair.

Remorse

What would it mean if someone hurt you, acknowledged what she had done, recognized the painful impact, and took responsibility for her actions—but then had no feelings of remorse for what she did? That person would seem insensitive and uncaring, if not spiteful or even cruel. Declaring and showing remorse are ways of saying, "It hurts me to know that I've put you through such pain. Your distress is now my distress—even more so because I'm the one who caused you to hurt." Remorse goes beyond accepting responsibility for hurting someone. To have remorse is to feel deep sadness, mourning, or even pain from the hurt you've brought to another person.

Restitution

When you do something wrong and hurt someone you love, often there's a desire to do something good to make up for the wrong or to make the bad feelings go away; these are acts of restitution. Although nothing can undo an affair, there are many things that someone can do to demonstrate feelings of remorse and perhaps reduce the distress of the injured partner. For example, in responding to Wendy's deep hurt from his affair, Ross told her:

> "I know that I can never make up for the terrible pain that I've caused you, and I will always feel horrible about that. But I will try as best I can to show you my commitment to our marriage by being less selfish and treating you more kindly. I know that it used to disappoint you that I spent much of my free time with my friends instead of with you, and I'm committed to changing that. I used to ignore your needs for a break from the kids and time with your own friends, and I'm determined to make sure you have at least one evening each week to spend with your friends. I can never undo what I did, but I can promise to do a better job of loving you."

It's important to distinguish between restitution and revenge. Restitution is an attempt by the offending partner to balance the scales by doing important *positive* things. By contrast, through revenge the injured person tries to balance the scales by retaliating with *negative* things toward the offending partner. Revenge may feel satisfying in the short run, but it rarely promotes healing in the long run.

As an injured partner, you need to examine the extent to which making amends is important for you to move forward. As a participating partner, it's important to recognize that moving on past the trauma of your affair will probably occur sooner or more fully when you work at caring for your partner's distress and nurturing your relationship. This is important to do even if the injured partner doesn't seem to acknowledge these efforts or doesn't respond in a positive way. You may have to persist at efforts to make restitution before things improve.

Reform

It's difficult to move beyond deep hurt unless you're assured that the person who caused you harm has committed not to hurt you in that way again.

>>> **Efforts by the participating partner toward reform include three steps:**
  1. **Pledging never to hurt your partner in the same way again.**
  2. **Addressing conditions that contributed to the affair.**
  3. **Acting differently when confronted with similar situations in the future.**

It's not realistic for partners to promise never to hurt one another at any level or in any form. But it *is* realistic to commit to avoiding certain hurtful behaviors—such as keeping secrets or engaging in inappropriate sexual or emotionally intimate relationships with others. Pursuing reform involves addressing and minimizing the contributing factors that you and your partner have identified that previously placed your relationship at risk for an affair. That includes not only addressing relationship issues such as levels of conflict or intimacy, but also continuing to work on individual issues (such as concerns about physical attractiveness or sexual adequacy) that contributed to having an affair. Promising to act differently is important to reform, but what's essential is actually *behaving* differently when temptations or opportunities for affairs arise. Evidence of reform helps to reestablish feelings of safety and trust that promote letting go of past hurt and moving on.

Release

"Release" comes closest to what we think of as the core of forgiveness. Release involves freeing both yourself and your partner from further punishment and domination by hurt or anger that lingers after the affair. Release doesn't mean approval; it doesn't require forgetting or no longer hurting. Rather, committing to release involves an explicit decision to work toward a process of moving on.

> Mario and Lila had worked together for almost a year to rebuild their marriage following Lila's affair. They had worked at examining and changing aspects of their relationship and themselves that had placed their marriage at risk. Both partners were clear about wanting to do whatever it took to save their marriage, but Mario continued to wrestle with memories of Lila's affair and the hurt and resentment toward Lila that these memories stirred up.
>
> "I can't just wipe the slate clean," he said in an individual therapy session. "It just doesn't feel right to me somehow, as if the affair never happened." Mario struggled with conflicting beliefs about forgiveness that were rooted in part in his religious upbringing. "I know we're supposed to forgive," he said. "But I also believe that on some level, even after we make confession and pledge to be different, we still carry the marks of our sins with us." Then he added, "I think I also relate 'wiping the slate clean' to 'forgetting it happened,' and I'm afraid that forgetting what happened could make us each more likely to slip back into the ways we interacted before Lila's affair that didn't work for us."
>
> Lila's remorse was evident to Mario, as were numerous ways in which she had worked to improve their marriage. Mario wrestled with his attitudes about forgiveness and read some books that helped him reflect more deeply on his religious beliefs. In a subsequent session he declared, "I think I've come to a decision about how to do this better. I can't wipe the slate clean; the affair happened and it can't be undone. But I can set that slate aside and start a new slate. The old slate won't just disappear, but I don't have to keep it out in the middle of our home anymore. I want us to write a new slate

together—that's what a fresh beginning means to me. Setting the old slate aside means we're removing it from being at the center of our lives and making the new slate our center."

Reconciliation

Recovery from an affair doesn't necessarily mean reconciling or staying in your marriage. Forgiveness doesn't require staying in an unhealthy relationship. In the next chapter, we're going to help you draw on everything you've learned and worked on to reach an explicit decision about how to move forward—either in this relationship or separately. But for some couples who work through the recovery process together—particularly those who follow a process similar to the one we've outlined in this book—reconciliation results from going through the previous steps we've described for moving on.

When Jeremy returned from an assignment overseas with his engineering firm, Marlene sensed that something was wrong. He was more quiet than usual and pulled back when she tried to cuddle with him. Their attempts at lovemaking during the first week after his return were brief and passionless, and Jeremy seemed distressed. After first denying that anything was wrong, he tearfully confessed that he had been sexually intimate with a consultant to their project whose home was abroad. He had no wish to continue his relationship with that woman at any level, but described feeling deeply confused about his feelings for Marlene. Jeremy felt tremendous remorse for his affair, but also wondered whether he could truly still love Marlene, given what he had done. His affair didn't make sense to either one of them.

Jeremy and Marlene spent several months examining the emotional distance that had grown between them in recent years. Both partners worked outside the home, and any free time had been devoted to their two daughters. Both also had substantial caretaking responsibilities for aging parents. Jeremy had never been good at recognizing or talking about his feelings with anyone, and this contributed to the gulf that had developed between him and Marlene.

Although clear from the beginning that they wanted to save their marriage, it was six months before Marlene was able to move beyond her deep hurt, and Jeremy beyond his own equally deep guilt, to be-

*come comfortable with each other and re-create an intimacy be-
tween them that had been missing for several years. They decided to
go away for a weekend without their daughters to one of their favorite places in the mountains, where they renewed their vows of commitment to one another. The ritual that Jeremy and Marlene created
symbolized their reconciliation and the promise of their new beginning.*

What Are the Barriers to Moving On?

Understanding the steps to moving on past deep relationship hurt can be
useful in understanding where you are in the process of recovering from
the affair. However, it's also important to understand some of the barriers
that can make this process more difficult.

Continued Hurtful Actions (or Inactions) of Your Partner

You may find it difficult to move on if your partner continues to behave in
ways that contribute to your feeling hurt or insecure in the relationship.
Your partner may continue to do things that used to be okay but that you
now find difficult to accept because of their association to the affair.
Maybe you didn't mind when your partner spent evenings out with
friends; but now the same types of evenings out make you uncomfortable,
if only because you've heard some of those friends making "jokes" about
"having some fun" outside marriage. No matter how innocent, trips out of
town, late nights at the office, or business lunches with members of the
opposite sex can easily trigger memories and feelings related to the affair.
And, of course, any continued contact with the outside person inevitably
stirs up continued apprehension, hurt, or resentment about the affair. The
bottom line is this: *What once may have been entirely innocent and "safe" behaviors may no longer be acceptable or may interfere with moving on because of
their association with the deeply painful affair.*

Both you and your partner need to examine carefully any potential
pitfalls along these lines so you can eliminate as many of them as possible.
But be realistic. Changing jobs or moving to a different community may
just not be possible. Completely cutting out all late evenings at work may
not be practical. Still, there are many ways of building in safety measures
that help to reduce anxieties and hurt feelings from the affair—such as

regularly checking in by phone when separated, arranging for other trusted workers of the same gender to be present when working late, or avoiding situations that unnecessarily stir up thoughts and feelings related to the affair.

Ultimately, you and your partner will need to collaborate in defining new arrangements that can be tolerated by both of you. These new limits or requirements won't work for your relationship if they're so harsh or punitive as to create resentment or push your partner away. But they may need to be more restrictive than before the affair—at least for a while—to help you in moving past the hurt.

Beliefs about Forgiveness

Read again through the list of common beliefs about forgiveness on page 277, and ask yourself whether any of these apply to you and whether they're making it more difficult for you to move on. For example, do you worry that if you let go of your hurt and became emotionally close to your partner, you might leave yourself open to being hurt by another affair? Or perhaps you sometimes worry that, by moving on past your hurt, your partner may believe you've come to accept what happened. Do you believe that expressing a commitment to move on would be tantamount to relinquishing your right to remember your partner's affair and feel hurt by those memories? Consider whether any of these beliefs are getting in the way of moving on and how you could think differently or adopt a different perspective that might work better for you. For example, if the idea of "wiping the slate clean" doesn't work for you, could you consider keeping that slate but setting it aside and then working with your partner toward writing a new one, as Mario did?

Fear of Being Hurt Again

The fear of another affair often provokes a constant state of vigilance, maintained in part by mentally rehearsing what happened in the past and all the factors that contributed to it. Constantly reliving the trauma of the affair keeps alive not just the memories but also the deep hurt feelings. We don't encourage you to stay in a relationship dominated by betrayals and mistrust. But "trust"—by definition—is different from "certainty." *Trust requires acting on faith without knowing for sure.*

You need to decide whether, based on everything you know about your partner and your marriage, you're willing to work toward rebuilding a relationship of mutual trust. If so, understand that doing so inevitably involves accepting some degree of risk of being hurt again—no matter how small. Holding on to your hurt won't eliminate that risk, and continuing either to retreat from or to lash out at your partner could eventually increase that risk.

Reluctance to Give Up Status as the Injured Party

Being the injured person provides an opportunity to claim the moral high ground by having been wronged. We've seen injured partners who have used their status as the offended person to maintain leverage in their relationship in demanding continued apologies, concessions, or reparations. We've also known injured partners who have used their hurt feelings from the affair as a reason for continuing to lash out and punish the participating partner long after the affair has ended. Letting go requires relinquishing the victim role and the benefits that go with it.

There's a fine line between requiring reform or restitution as a basis for moving on past hurt feelings, and using hurt feelings as a way of maintaining influence or inflicting further hurt in a relationship. If you're having difficulty letting go, consider whether any part of your difficulty relates to advantages in the relationship you might need to give up by deciding to forgive or move on.

How Do I Get Unstuck?

If you're still having difficulty moving beyond intense hurt and anger left over from your partner's affair, pursue the additional steps described below.

Evaluate the Risks and Benefits of Moving On

The primary risk of moving on is opening yourself to being hurt again. But you may also end up disappointed by an expectation that you'll never have any hurt feelings related to the affair. And what might happen when you relinquish the extra influence you've had in the relationship simply by being recognized by your partner as the injured party? These may feel like significant risks to you, but the relationship risks of not moving on are equal or greater. Continued domination of a relationship through righteous hurt or anger will eventually destroy any opportunity to rebuild a healthy relationship. Fostering feelings of guilt in your partner by holding on to your own hurt or anger will eventually change guilt into resentment.

By contrast, when you want your relationship to succeed and you want to care for your partner's well-being, letting go of past hurt often serves as a powerful gift that not only promotes better emotional and physical health in both of you but frequently inspires your partner to work harder on behalf of the relationship and give more in return.

Make a Decision to Forgive or Move On

In his book *Forgiveness Is a Choice*, Robert Enright emphasizes that letting go of one's hurt and forgiving the wrongdoer are choices that one is free to either accept or reject. The decision to forgive doesn't mean that you've completed the process, but rather that you've made "a good beginning" in committing to the process. Making a decision to let go of hurt and anger requires carefully evaluating the strategies you've used for moving on so far and how those strategies have either helped or fallen short. To decide to move on, you have to have a vision of how you want to be emotionally, relationally, and perhaps spiritually—and commit to a process that has greater potential to get you there. Exercise 12.2 can help you in this process.

You may still have difficulty disrupting negative thoughts and feelings related to the affair even after reaching a decision to forgive or let go of the hurt. If you find yourself in this situation, the following guidelines may help.

• *Find more constructive ways of venting your feelings.* Although sometimes it may be important to share your hurt feelings with your partner (for example, explaining that you need some time by yourself before you can resume interacting in a warm or intimate way), it's also important that you have ways of expressing your feelings separately from your partner. Alternative ways of venting your feelings include keeping a journal or sharing your feelings with a trusted friend, keeping in mind the guidelines for this included in Chapter 4.

• *Work toward developing more effective techniques for managing your feelings when they threaten to escalate out of control.* Be sure to recognize when your feelings may be getting out of control—such as when you're having particularly "hot thoughts," having muscle tightness or other physical signs of tension, speaking in a harsh or angry manner, slamming doors, or experiencing other cues of escalating anger that you've learned to recognize. Use some of the techniques for managing intense feelings outlined in Chapter 3—using meditation or relaxation, going for a walk, engaging in moderate exercise, or taking a time-out until your feelings are under better control.

• *Develop more effective techniques for disrupting negative thoughts that interfere with more positive feelings or constructive behaviors.* Recognizing repetitive negative thoughts and simply telling yourself to "stop" can sometimes be helpful, as can limiting your time for having such thoughts to a particular time of day or set period (for example, for 15 minutes but not longer). Redirecting your thoughts to a different topic or distracting yourself by engaging in a different activity can also help. Another way of disrupting negative thoughts is to think about things from a different, more positive perspective. For example, rather than focusing on your disappointment that you continue to have memories of your partner's affair, remind yourself that the memories don't occur nearly as often or that the hurt feelings aren't as devastating or as long lasting as they once were. Participating partners, too, can remind themselves, when dismayed about still harboring memories or feelings of nostalgia for the affair, of the progress already made toward taking responsibility and pursuing reform.

• *Work toward developing compassion for your partner.* First you have to develop an understanding of how your partner came to act in a hurtful way and recognize your partner's own distress. The work you've already done in Chapters 7 through 11 should help you develop this understanding and empathy for your partner's experience. Compassion comes from caring for your partner and wishing an end to your partner's own pain— whether you're the injured partner or the partner who participated in the affair.

• *Draw on spiritual or similar resources that help to provide meaning in letting go and strengthen your efforts toward this goal.* If feeling hurt or angry interferes with your efforts to let go of the past for the sake of your partner or your relationship, you can still work toward forgiveness based on personal or spiritual values. From this perspective, the benefits of moving on go beyond personal or relationship consequences and involve the inherent goodness or "rightness" of forgiving someone who has wronged you. Drawing on personal or spiritual values can help you work toward letting go of the past even when you don't feel like doing so. If you're the participating partner, see the following section, where we discuss how you can try to forgive yourself and let go as well.

- *Express your desire to forgive or move on and describe steps you're willing to take toward this process.* Making an explicit declaration to your partner about your commitment to moving on can promote greater understanding and patience from your partner when you experience setbacks in letting go and may help your partner with letting go of hurt or resentment from the past as well. It's important that you both understand that your commitment to moving on implies a process that is still unfolding, not an end state that has already been achieved. It doesn't mean you won't continue to remember or hurt from the affair. It means you no longer allow hurt or anger to rule your life and you relinquish your right to continue punishing your partner or demanding further restitution.

For Participating Partners: How Do I Forgive Myself?

Participating partners often struggle with issues of forgiveness, particularly forgiving themselves for an affair. For example, you may fear that forgiving yourself would make it easier to forget what happened and let down your guard against hurting your partner again. You may be reluctant to seek your partner's forgiveness because you believe doing so would imply seeking pardon or acceptance for what you did. Your compassion for your partner's continued hurt may make it difficult for you to move beyond your guilt and shame—or may lead to a sense that you need to continue suffering at least as long as your partner suffers. (Injured partners also may wrestle with forgiving themselves for their own roles that made their relationship more vulnerable, or for some of their hurtful or punitive responses to the affair that damaged the relationship even further.)

The consequences of not forgiving yourself for what you did related to the affair are the same as for not forgiving someone else. In the short run, appropriate levels of guilt can help to motivate and sustain changes in your own behavior that are difficult to make. But excessive guilt or shame tends to immobilize people and prevent constructive changes from occurring.

Not just for your own sake, but for your partner's and your relationship's sake, it's important to examine whether you may need to forgive yourself. If you're struggling with self-forgiveness, we encourage you to read through the guidelines outlined in this chapter and apply them to letting go of shame or anger you have toward yourself. Consider factors that could be keeping you stuck—including beliefs about forgiveness, actions (or inactions) of your partner, or advantages you may be reluctant to give up by holding on to your guilt (for example, lessening your partner's wish to punish you or seek further restitution). Consider also the risks of not forgiving yourself and moving on. What specific steps toward implementing a decision to forgive yourself are you willing to commit to? How could these be helpful not only to you, but also to your relationship?

What's Next?

Work through the following exercises, which will help you to examine where you are currently in the process of moving on and then to reach and implement a decision to let go of the hurt and anger that continue to damage you or your relationship. Chapter 13 will then help you reach an explicit decision about how to move forward—either by staying in this relationship or by moving on separately.

———————————— Exercises ————————————

EXERCISE 12.1. EXAMINING YOUR PROGRESS TOWARD MOVING ON

Moving on isn't a single step but a process or a series of steps. This exercise guides you in evaluating how far you and your partner have come in terms of moving on past the affair. *Make two lists.*

First, what steps have you and your partner already accomplished in moving on? What has each of you done to make things better? For example, you might recognize that your partner has taken full responsibility for the affair and is behaving much more appropriately around those of the opposite sex. Or perhaps you realize that earlier you took every opportunity to hurt your partner with painful reminders of the affair, but you now try to avoid doing this.

Second, make a list of the steps you still need to take to move forward and clarify the barriers that are making these difficult or holding you back. What would you need to do to overcome these barriers? How could your partner be helpful? For example, you might realize that you need to start demonstrating some level of trust in your partner not to betray you again. In spite of your fear that you could be hurt again, you may need to decide on reasonable limits for your partner's behavior and then give your partner a chance to be faithful to you. Or perhaps you or your partner have begun to engage in behaviors that previously put your relationship at risk—for example, devoting long hours to work or other activities outside the home and neglecting your relationship when together. If you or your partner recognize this as a barrier to moving on, you need to work toward establishing or renewing healthier limits on outside involvements and better ways of connecting with each other.

EXERCISE 12.2.
REACHING A DECISION TO LET GO OF THE HURT OR ANGER

First, list the potential risks and benefits of letting go of your hurt or angry feelings. Then list the benefits and risks of not letting go. For example, as the injured partner, you might believe your anger is one of the main things that motivates your partner to change, and if you let go of it, your partner will go back to his or her old ways. At the same time, you know that, in the long run, a strong relationship needs to be based on love, not anger. Or as the participating partner, you might believe, *"I've hurt my partner horribly, and I deserve to suffer for it. Every day I need to remind myself of what I've done."* Although accepting responsibility and committing to change are critical to healing, daily doses of guilt and self-punishment for the rest of your life will beat you down, which helps neither you nor your partner.

Second, consider strategies you can implement if you continue to feel stuck in your hurt or anger despite your decision to move on. Negative feelings often continue long term because they're related to how you think about things. For example, if you continue to dwell on each instance when your partner lied to you in order to be with the other person, going over these events from the past is likely to keep your anger alive by reminding you how you were mistreated and deceived. Therefore, focusing your thoughts instead on your partner's positive efforts to improve your relationship once the affair ended might reduce your hurt or anger.

Or instead of going over and over your partner's faults and flaws, you might pursue ways of developing some compassion for your partner. For example, you might conclude:

"It's not an excuse, but I know you're imperfect, with shortcomings like everyone else. You grew up in a family where you didn't learn from your parents how to be committed when things get tough between people. I know you get frightened and insecure when things aren't going well between us, and that vulnerability is part of what attracted me to you. So I want to care for you and hold you when you feel frightened, but I can't do that if you betray me."

Stepping back and taking a broader perspective on the betrayal may encourage more understanding and feelings of empathy toward your partner.

13

Can This Marriage Be Saved?

Neil and Rhonda had been struggling for six months to recover from Rhonda's affair with Neil's best friend. Rhonda had told Neil about the affair and had agreed to end it, but Neil continued to wrestle with the pains of betrayal by both Rhonda and his friend. Rhonda had been close to moving out of their home before her affair, following almost a year of frequent marital conflicts and mutual retreat from each other. The couple's efforts to cope with Rhonda's affair and to understand everything that had gone wrong began as a last-ditch effort to determine whether their marriage could be saved.

They had lots of reasons to try to make it work. For the most part, they were well matched, with similar values and personalities. Both were devoted parents to their 8-year-old son, and they worked hard to balance their home life with their respective jobs. Following the initial chaos that accompanied Rhonda's disclosure of her affair and her moving out for two weeks to stay with a friend, they had committed to examining how the affair happened and what it would take to restore their marriage. It wasn't difficult to identify various stressors that had come between them. Rhonda recognized deep feelings of loneliness and resentment toward her in-laws, which she had been reluctant to express to Neil before her affair. With time, Neil also came to understand that by throwing himself into endless projects helping his parents out on their farm, he had neglected both his and Rhonda's needs for emotional closeness.

Over the past six months, they had made lots of progress in talk-

ing about their feelings and making better decisions about how to spend their time together at home. It had taken a while before Neil started to warm up again, but Rhonda had been patient. Eventually Neil no longer had the same deep bitterness toward Rhonda he had felt initially, and at times things between them seemed back to normal.

Still, some of the hurtful consequences of Rhonda's affair continued. For Neil, something in their relationship seemed lost forever. He could no longer view Rhonda in the same way. He had once felt completely comfortable with her in a way he had never experienced with any other woman. Now when Rhonda wasn't at home, he couldn't help thinking of her affair and getting that knot in his stomach. He and Rhonda had restored a decent friendship, but the laughter and delight they had once enjoyed with each other hadn't returned.

Neil didn't want to end his marriage, but he also didn't want to spend the rest of his life in a marriage that lacked real intimacy or passion. Would those feelings of trust ever come back? How long would it take? If they never came back, would he be able to accept that but keep his marriage? Or would he and Rhonda be better off ending their marriage as friends and moving on separately?

Some couples, like Neil and Rhonda, work hard to understand the affair and restore a caring relationship but continue to struggle to recapture feelings of trust, intimacy, or joy with each other. Even after getting beyond the intense anger related to the affair, deciding whether to move on together or separately can be difficult. In this chapter we'll help you arrive at an explicit decision about how to move forward—either by staying with your partner and recommitting to your relationship or by moving on separately. Exercise 13.1 will guide you toward this decision, and Exercise 13.2 will help you identify specific steps for implementing it. You may already have decided how to move forward. If so, we still encourage you to read this chapter and work through the exercises. Doing so may help you form clearer reasons for your decision or help you discuss this decision with your partner more effectively. Examining the issues considered here may also help you anticipate work that you or your partner may still need to pursue either to help your marriage succeed or to lead fulfilling lives separately.

What Are My Choices?

Following an affair, some people know immediately that they're both willing and able to recommit to their marriages. Others choose at the outset to separate from their partners and work toward divorce. Most people, however—particularly injured partners—have mixed feelings. Many would like their marriages to work but feel too frightened, hurt, or angry to know if this is possible. Others lean toward separation, but don't want to give up on their relationships without first making every possible effort to reconcile. Ultimately, the paths for moving forward fall into four types:

1. Moving on together in a healthy way. Some couples commit to rebuilding their marriages and do the work needed to make this happen. Both partners work to manage their own feelings of hurt, anger, shame, or doubt in ways that are least damaging and permit positive steps forward to continue. Both partners work to restore trust and emotional intimacy. The affair isn't forgotten, but it serves as a reminder of the need to continually nurture and strengthen the relationship and deal with stresses or conflicts as they arise.

2. Moving on together in an unhealthy way. Couples sometimes stay together following a partner's affair but do so poorly. They continue to interact in hurtful ways—damaging each other's relationships with their children or with others, having frequent or intense arguments, or failing to reestablish a positive relationship. One or both partners may continue to violate agreements regarding relationships with others. If not actively hurtful in their exchanges, partners remain isolated in emotional retreat. Either partner may privately wish for the marriage to end. Persistent deep feelings of hurt, anger, or mistrust block necessary steps toward restoring a constructive and intimate relationship.

3. Moving on separately in a healthy way. Partners end their relationship in a way that is least hurtful to themselves and to others they love, including their children and extended families. They work hard not to inflict further damage on each other during the process of separation or divorce. If they have children, they work together to protect the emotional and physical well-being of those children in both the short and long terms. They let go of their anger and resolve not to punish each other further. They each use what they've learned from the affair to establish happy and productive lives, either alone or in a healthy relationship with someone new.

4. Moving on separately in an unhealthy way. Partners separate and may divorce, but they continue to interact in hurtful ways. Similar to those who stay together in unhealthy ways, they damage each other's relationships with their children, respective families, or friends and colleagues. They continue to argue over money or property. Or they cut off all further contact but continue to relive conflicts from their relationship or trauma related to the affair in their minds. Their lingering bitterness or wounded feelings often interfere with forming healthy new intimate relationships and can have a lasting negative impact on their children's intimate relationships as well.

Of course, no one actively seeks the unhealthy options. But some people end up there by default—by failing to choose and commit to the healthier alternatives. Moving on in a healthy way, either together or separately, requires you to carefully evaluate the resources and potential risks that you each bring to your relationship, decide to stay together or not, and then commit to implementing that decision as positively as possible.

How Do I Decide?

It's not uncommon for people to have mixed feelings about their relationship, particularly when they've experienced frequent or intense arguing or gone through long periods of loneliness or emotional withdrawal. After an affair, mixed feelings are more often the norm than the exception. It may be that no decision you reach about your relationship will feel absolutely certain to you. As we've said earlier, if you wait to be completely sure that your marriage will work before committing to it, you probably won't be able to begin or continue with the difficult efforts that are required to make your marriage succeed. Similarly, if you wait to be completely sure that ending your marriage will ultimately provide a healthier and more fulfilling life, you may end up staying in an unhealthy relationship that continues to be hurtful or emotionally empty.

It's important to struggle through your mixed feelings and try to reach a decision to move forward in one direction or the other. Evaluating what you've learned about your partner, your relationship, and yourself is vital to reaching the right decision.

Evaluating Your Partner

Think back to aspects of your partner that you considered in working through the chapters in Part II. If you're the injured person, what did you conclude about your partner's character? Was your partner's affair an isolated event or, instead, part of a long series of betrayals? Perhaps your partner engaged in the affair during a time of serious relationship problems. Or maybe the affair resulted from your partner's underlying attitude of "entitlement" or a pattern of acting impulsively without regard for the feelings of others. Did the affair stem in part from positive aspects of your partner—including emotional sensitivity or needs for connection?

Has your partner accepted responsibility for the affair and expressed genuine remorse? Has your partner demonstrated the ability to make difficult changes in the past—including changes unrelated to your relationship? Consider whether your partner has implemented important changes since the affair. For example, if a contributing factor to the affair was your partner's spending time in situations that encouraged flirtatious or intimate behavior, has he committed to avoiding such circumstances? Similarly, if your partner's vulnerability to an affair included difficulty in expressing feelings or needs in the marriage, has he worked to convey these more effectively? Has your partner addressed outside factors that increased vulnerability to an affair? For example, has he limited time at work or with friends that detracted from intimacy in your relationship? Have your partner's interactions with the outside affair person been eliminated entirely or restricted to those absolutely essential because of a shared work setting?

If you're the participating partner struggling with a decision about how to move forward, evaluating factors involving your partner is equally important. For example, has your partner been willing to examine his own contributions to your relationship that may have placed it at greater risk for an affair? Has your partner reached a decision to work past deep hurt or anger from your affair, and has he shown progress in this direction? In considering these questions, it's important to remember that injured partners typically require a much longer time to recover from an affair than participating partners. You may be struggling to decide for yourself whether to stay in your marriage well before your partner is able to consider such a decision. If that's so, then our best advice is to remain patient for now and to focus on how to move forward within the marriage as best you can until you're fairly certain that either (1) your injured partner won't be able to restore a positive or close relationship with you regardless of time and efforts, or (2) regardless of your partner's decision about the marriage and ability to recover, you want to end the relationship and move on separately.

Evaluating Your Relationship

Review the factors in your relationship you identified previously that potentially increased its vulnerability to an affair. To what extent have you and your partner addressed these concerns? If you previously had frequent or intense conflicts, have you developed more effective strategies for managing your differences and reaching decisions together? Consider whether you've been able to resolve specific areas of disagreement—for example, for dealing with finances, children, or leisure time. If your relationship suffered from differences in expectations or frustrations from responsibilities in or outside the home, have you redefined roles in ways that reduce these tensions or bring greater satisfaction to you both? If your relationship became vulnerable partly because of feeling disconnected from each other, have you found more effective ways to promote emotional or physical intimacy?

Even if your marriage prior to the affair was mostly satisfying for you both, the trauma of the affair almost certainly caused significant stress to your relationship and may have produced lingering negative effects. Have you and your partner been able to avoid damaging interactions following the affair? If the affair created new problems in your relationship—for example, conflicts with in-laws or inability to make unified decisions about finances or the children—consider whether you've been able to work together to resolve them. Have you found ways to laugh together or do some of the things you used to enjoy as a couple? If negative interactions related to the affair continue, have you at least managed to reduce their frequency and intensity? Do you and your partner share a common vision of how you'd like to move forward as a couple?

In addition, think about your relationship from the larger perspective. Why did you and your partner decide to become a couple, and how has your relationship helped you grow? Consider what you've done best together and what challenges you've overcome. Before the affair, was there more good in this marriage than bad? If so, can you recover what once was mostly good?

Evaluating Yourself

As the injured partner, you'll need to address several challenges in order to move forward in this relationship in a healthy way. First, you need to find ways to manage your feelings so that you don't continue to lash out destructively at your partner or become overwhelmed with feelings of despair. Second, you need to examine aspects of yourself that may have contributed to your relationship's becoming vulnerable to an affair. For example, if difficulties in managing your anger contributed to intense arguments or retreat by your partner, you need to develop more effective self-control. Or if your discomfort with vulnerable feelings contributed to emotional distance between the two of you, you need to develop ways of tolerating and discussing such feelings. Third, regardless of your decision to stay in this relationship or not, it's important that you find ways to move past your deep hurt to focus on the life ahead of you. Finally, if you decide to stay in this relationship, it will be important to rediscover or promote new ways of pursuing joy and intimacy with your partner. It won't be enough for you or your partner simply to stop arguing; vital relationships require more. Are you willing to take gradual, appropriate risks in restoring trust in your partner and intimacy in your relationship?

If you're the participating partner, you have challenges of your own to address in deciding how to move forward. Do you want to save your marriage? If so, have you honestly examined aspects of yourself that led to your affair? Have you identified and addressed your own contributions to vulnerabilities in this relationship? Consider what you're willing to give, and what you'll give up, to help your marriage succeed. Can you commit to making your marriage work in the long term even if your injured partner is struggling with this in the short term? You may need to let go of your own hurt feelings from the marriage or your partner's behaviors either prior to or following the affair. If guilt or shame is interfering with your ability to restore an intimate and joyful relationship with your partner, are you prepared to do whatever it takes to move past those feelings?

Additional Considerations

Concerns about the potential impact of divorce on children influence many people's decisions about whether to stay together. What that impact might be is very difficult to predict. A wide range of studies have researched the question and come up with conflicting results. Professionals disagree enormously about the effects of marital conflict and divorce on children. One thing that is clear, however, is that many different factors come into play, from the quality of the parents' relationship and parent–child interactions before divorce, to the children's ages, postdivorce involvement with their parents and the parents' interactions with each other, and how the divorce affects the children's economic and social well-being. It's also clear that deciding not to divorce "for the sake of the children" rarely serves them well if their parents continue to have frequent and intense arguments. *So, we're left with the indisputable conclusion that children's overall emotional well-being is best served when their parents either*:

- Reduce the frequency and intensity of arguments in the home—particularly those witnessed by their children; or
- Collaborate as parents and minimize continuing conflicts following separation or divorce.

The implication is obvious: Whether you decide to move forward together or separately, commit to moving on in a healthy way for the sake of your children.

For some people, the decision about whether to stay in a marriage is also strongly influenced by personal or religious values. We wouldn't presume to address these influences here, other than to urge you to recognize the potential importance of this factor in your decision. If you're struggling with such issues, seek spiritual direction from a trusted spiritual adviser.

You may also find it useful to talk with carefully selected friends, family members, or professional counselors, but with family members or friends, set limits on how much you'll disclose (see Chapter 4). Most important, be careful about placing too much weight on any advice you receive, no matter how well intended. Ultimately, you need to take ownership and responsibility for reaching and implementing your own decision.

Talk with your partner about factors you're considering as you work toward a decision, and invite your partner's own evaluations. Begin by reviewing positive reasons for staying in the relationship and for continuing your work toward making it better. Then identify remaining concerns and describe their importance. What would it take from each of you to address them? Talking with your partner about whether to continue your relationship will likely be very difficult, so be sure to use the strategies described in Chapter 3 for managing strong negative feelings that may arise during this discussion.

Finally, remember that ultimately it will require work from both of you to make your relationship succeed. Either one of you can end the relationship regardless of the other one's wishes or efforts. Similarly, either of you can undermine or sabotage the relationship by letting your partner do all the work of changing.

What If I Decide to Stay?

If you've been working through this book largely on your own, now is a good time to invite your partner again to read through the book and work with you. You may not both need to complete all the exercises at this time. But even if you've already worked through them by yourself, your partner should join you in identifying what put your relationship at risk and addressing these factors as fully as possible.

Beyond that, if you and your partner decide to move forward together, your challenge will be to continue the efforts you began as you worked through the earlier chapters—healing the past, strengthening the present, and enriching the future. The kinds of work required have already been introduced, but certain aspects of this work, described below, will require continued effort.

Healing the Past

You began work aimed at healing the past when you and your partner first had discussions about what happened and how it impacted you both. Disclosing difficult feelings to each other and acknowledging them in a caring way may be the most critical steps toward moving beyond deep hurt from the affair. It's vital that the participating partner state with conviction, in words of his or her own choosing, "I know what I did was horribly wrong, and I'm profoundly sorry. I can't undo what I've done, but I'll do everything I can to make our relationship right."

To move forward together, it's important that you as the injured partner accept this apology—not by excusing the affair or agreeing never to feel hurt or angry about what happened but simply by acknowledging the apology and your partner's pledge to reform. It's also important to commit to a process of releasing your partner from further punishment. It won't be possible to heal the past if your relationship continues to be dominated by guilt, shame, or retribution.

Healing from an affair requires you to develop the best understanding possible of how the affair came about. However, there comes a point at which no further discussion is likely to provide new information or promote deeper understanding. If you and your partner have already reached that point, further cycling through questions of "Why did you do it?" will feel exhausting and may interfere with reestablishing closeness and moving on together. Does the information you have so far about why the affair occurred give you and your partner guidance about what you each need to do differently? If so, it may be time to let go of further questions about "why" the affair occurred to focus instead on rebuilding the future.

Finally, it's important to remember that healing from the past is a process that will likely continue even after you've worked through issues of forgiveness or letting go and reached a clear decision to move forward together. There will be times in the future when you or your partner remember the affair and its impact with feelings of hurt, sadness, or resentment. At those times, try to focus on how far you've already come in the healing process, regain your vision of where you and your partner want to be in the future, and recommit to doing what it takes in the moment to tolerate or work beyond those feelings.

Strengthening the Present

In previous chapters we repeatedly encouraged you to consider what it would take to reduce the risk factors in your marriage and increase the protective factors—in you, your partner, and your relationship. Review your responses to the exercises in those chapters. Have you identified sources of conflict and developed better strategies for managing differences? Have you restored emotional and physical intimacy? What about risks from outside your marriage? How are you drawing on others to support your marriage? Review how you've addressed aspects of yourselves that placed your marriage at risk for an affair. Have you strengthened aspects of yourselves that are essential to recovery?

Strengthening the present doesn't mean trying to get back to where you were; it means making the most of where you are. It involves more than reducing conflict and requires creating opportunities for intimacy and joy. It requires implementing everything you've learned about maintaining a secure and loving relationship and continuing in those efforts, especially when it's difficult and you may least feel like doing so.

Enriching the Future

Couples can stay together but remain stuck. Moving forward requires a vision of where you want to be and a road map for getting there. On one level, the road map may involve specific plans for dealing with setbacks and getting back on track. For example, it may be important to anticipate how to remain connected when either one of you experiences difficult feelings in response to seeing an affair portrayed in the movies or by attending a wedding and witnessing vows of fidelity. On another level, moving forward involves envisioning the bigger picture of your long-term future together. You and your partner will feel more emotionally connected when you share a vision of how you want to develop as a couple or family. Talk with your partner about your dreams of how you'd like to move forward and what you're willing to do to make your dreams a reality.

How Do I Regain Trust?

Trust can be one of the last important qualities to return to a committed relationship after an affair. Some people struggle with this more than others because they were wounded or betrayed in previous relationships. Some people struggle more with earning or maintaining trust because of tendencies to be secretive or to test the boundaries of relationship rules or expectations. By and large, most couples enter committed relationships or marriage with high levels of mutual trust. However, once an affair has occurred, trust can be extraordinarily difficult to recover. Rebuilding trust takes time, and progress along the way often requires small, incremental steps.

It's helpful to distinguish among different levels or kinds of trust. Apart from issues of fidelity, you or your partner may have concerns about trust regarding specific issues or areas in your relationship. For example, can you trust your partner to listen when you're discussing an issue? Can you trust your partner to treat you with courtesy and respect when you're around others? Can your partner be trusted to honor agreements you've made about managing money? If you tell your partner you'll be home at a given time, can she count on you to show up then or to call ahead of time? Can your partner trust you to set aside time to be together when work demands increase? One way to work toward rebuilding trust is to co-operate in reaching and keeping agreements on specific issues or in partic-ular areas one at a time. As trust grows in specific areas, this often creates a sense of hope and begins to rebuild feelings of trust on a more general level as well.

Efforts to regain trust include the following:

- As the injured partner:
  —Taking small gradual risks and tolerating initial discomfort.
- As the participating partner:
  —Eliminating secrecy.
  —Honoring relationship boundaries.
  —Keeping agreements with your partner about specific issues in your rela-tionship.

Rebuilding Trust When You're the Injured Partner

You need to decide whether you're willing to work toward rebuilding a re-lationship of mutual trust. Doing so inevitably involves accepting some degree of risk of being hurt again—no matter how small. Rebuilding trust doesn't require no longer worrying; instead, it involves identifying gradual risks you're willing to take and your ability to tolerate the discomfort of never knowing for certain that you couldn't be betrayed again. Talk with your partner about your fears. When are the times you feel least secure? Which risk factors do you feel least confident about having eliminated? Discuss additional steps you could take to reduce those risks. For example, does your partner continue in certain activities away from home that you previously identified as potential risks? What could your partner say or do differently at those times to reassure you?

Think about the different situations that contribute to your feeling mistrustful or uncertain of your partner's pledge to remain faithful. List these situations in order of difficulty—from those that trigger only low levels of apprehension to those that trigger the highest. For example, when your partner comes home from work but appears quiet or with-drawn, you may wonder whether your partner has run into the outside af-fair person who works at the same office. Your discomfort may be only slight, and your partner's willingness to talk about what happened during the day or simply tell you whether there's been any contact with the outside person (and the nature of that contact) may reassure you. However, if your partner is working late at night but doesn't call or can't be reached by phone, your worry about your partner's continuing involvement with the outside person may be considerably greater and reassurances after your partner gets home may not be enough. In that case, the two of you may need to agree on how late to stay at work, how to stay connected by phone while physically apart, and who else needs to be present for you not to worry about inappropriate behaviors.

What are the smallest steps you're willing to take now toward reestablishing trust? Consider working toward specific agreements with your partner around issues separate from fidelity. For example, would it help to rebuild trust if your partner kept agreements about spending time with you or the children instead of at work or with others? Would your relationship feel more secure if your partner talked with you about hurt feelings or decisions you're both facing in your relationship? Following through on such commitments may not eliminate your trust issues around fidelity—but these efforts can provide an initial foundation for rebuilding trust on a more general level.

Separate from your partner's efforts, what will you have to do on your own to tolerate discomfort in accepting some risk, no matter how small? For example, would it help to remind yourself of your partner's efforts when you're struggling with feelings of mistrust? What would be some indicators along the way that you were making progress in rebuilding trust? For example, worries about what your partner is doing when you're apart might occur less frequently, be less intense, or be put to rest more easily after seeking information or reassurance. While trying to rebuild trust, recognize that this will take time. Look for opportunities to move forward in small increments. If you continue to have difficulty in working toward a trusting relationship, review the discussion in Chapter 12 regarding barriers to moving on and strategies for getting unstuck.

Regaining Your Partner's Trust after You've Had an Affair

Taking responsibility for the affair and promising to change are necessary but usually not enough to regain your partner's trust. Being faithful now doesn't prove that you won't be unfaithful down the road. To regain your partner's trust, you have to commit to reform in the ways described in

Chapter 12 and then take steps to go beyond these essentials. For example, it's not enough not to keep secrets; you need to work at being completely open, particularly in terms of your interactions with the outside affair partner or anyone else your partner may regard as a potential threat. Not only is it important not to engage in emotional or physical intimacy with anyone other than your partner, you need to adhere to tighter boundaries that show that you won't even get close to having a special relationship with someone else. Remember that your partner may no longer be able or willing to accept some of your behaviors that were okay in the past—for example, spending time away from home by yourself or with friends—because those behaviors serve as reminders of a whole range of risk factors that may have contributed to your affair.

You may have found it easier to accept restrictions or tolerate your partner's mistrust earlier, when your partner first learned of your affair, but now find it increasingly difficult to deal with your partner's continuing mistrust. Talk with your partner about the times you experience his or her mistrust. Explore ways in which you can meet your partner's increased needs for security while working toward small steps of rebuilding trust. Remember that your partner's ability to trust you will probably develop more slowly than your need to receive that trust.

Begin rebuilding trust by identifying specific concerns your partner has and then reaching agreements together about behaviors you're willing and able to perform. For example, if you've pledged to be more helpful around the house, develop a list together of what you'll do specifically to help and when or how often you'll do this. If you've promised to spend more time together, talk with your partner about specific shared activities that demonstrate your commitment to building a close relationship—and then take initiative for making those activities happen.

Barry's affair occurred after six months of Robyn's spending most weeks on the opposite coast opening a branch store for her corporation. While Robyn was gone, Barry had been invited to dinner on several occasions by Eve, a recently divorced colleague at his office. Barry found himself drawn to Eve but was uneasy with his feelings and consistently declined her invitations. However, on one occasion when Robyn had been gone for nearly a month, he accepted Eve's invitation for dinner at her home and they subsequently spent the night together. In the following days, Barry couldn't make sense of his feelings. The encounter with Eve felt simultaneously exhilarating and horribly wrong.

Barry confessed the incident to Robyn several weeks after she returned. In the difficult months that followed, they identified numerous factors in and around their marriage that had made it vulnerable to an affair. Both partners wanted to salvage their marriage if possible, and they rapidly moved to place limits on outside intrusions and set aside time for themselves. Barry grappled with a lifelong difficulty in expressing his feelings—a handicap that left Robyn feeling bewildered about why he sometimes seemed unhappy or frustrated with her. Separately Robyn struggled to overcome insecurities that had played havoc with their relationship from the beginning, particularly in terms of her jealousy over any interactions Barry had with women at work—even those in public or group settings.

Regaining trust required special efforts by both partners. Barry recognized that, given both Robyn's insecurities and the night he had spent with Eve, he needed to be completely open with Robyn about any interactions with others even if this sometimes caused her to feel more distressed. He went to considerable lengths to keep her informed of where he was during the day, whether he needed to work late, and—if so—who else would be there with him. Robyn also worked to understand her own insecurities better and to identify reasons for feeling more confident in herself. She worked toward decreasing the frequent reassurances she needed from Barry. Her next assignment away from home renewed her insecurities and presented the couple with difficult challenges, but also opportunities to identify better ways of staying connected during Robyn's absences and communicating about their needs for each other.

Within a year after Barry's affair, they had restored their relationship and, by addressing previous risk factors, had created a healthier and more resilient marriage together.

What If I Decide to Leave?

If either one of you decides to end your relationship, how you implement that decision will influence not only how constructive or damaging the process is, but potentially also how well you move forward after the separation or divorce is complete.

Moving on separately in a healthy way requires two things from you and your partner:

1. Anticipating practical and emotional issues for you and others directly affected by this decision.
2. Maintaining your dignity by treating each other with courtesy and civility.

The latter may seem undeserved by your partner and may require extraordinary effort on your part, but the long-term benefits of maintaining your self-respect by behaving civilly during this difficult process are well worth the struggle.

What Will I Need to Plan For?

The list of items to consider when pursuing separation or divorce is potentially endless, but broad themes include pragmatic concerns related to living arrangements, finances, division of property, and informing others. Special themes that we'll consider separately include how to care for your children and how to care for yourself.

If possible, it's important for you and your partner to discuss where each of you will live in the short term during the separation process and in the longer term once the separation or divorce is complete. Some couples manage to stay in the same house through part or most of the initial process, working together to sort through financial issues or prepare their home for sale. More often, one partner finds a place to live temporarily until more permanent arrangements can be made. If separating, determine who will be responsible for which bills until the divorce is finalized—including house or car payments, credit card debts, clothing or medical expenses for the children, and so on. You may need to evaluate your own work situation and ensure that you will have adequate income once your relationship ends. Initial discussions about shared property may be useful, particularly as these relate to major purchases you might face when setting up separate households. You may also need to discuss how to divide assets that have special emotional meaning or how to divide or share pets. Avoid arguing over "pots and pans"—relatively small items of little emotional value that can easily be replaced. Try to use the decision-making skills described in Chapter 3, and use time-outs if necessary to disrupt unproductive negative exchanges.

There are numerous self-help books and resources on the Internet regarding how to pursue a constructive divorce. We've listed a few of these in the "Additional Resources" section at the end of this book. If you and your partner have managed to maintain a cooperative relationship, you may be able to work toward separation or divorce largely on your own or with the help of a mediator without the costs or stress of hiring separate attorneys in an adversarial process. A financial planner may also be helpful in sorting through complicated retirement funds or other investments, as well as planning for items such as children's college expenses.

At some point you'll need to inform others of your decision to end your relationship. It's best to work through that process slowly, beginning with those who most need to know (for example, members of your family or your employer). Avoid going into detail about the struggles you and your partner have had. Talking about your partner in negative ways can place friends or even family members in a difficult position, and down the road you and your partner may want to interact together with these people at large family events like graduations, weddings, or funerals. Ask friends and family to honor your decision and, if possible, invite them to maintain a separate relationship with your partner if they would like.

How Should We Care for Our Children?

Numerous resources are available on how to help your children through separation or divorce, both in bookstores and on the Internet. We've listed some of these in the section on resources as well. Basically, the principles to follow are similar to those described in Chapter 4. *Specifically, place your children's well-being above your own hurt and anger.* Of course, that's easier said than done. The best way to ensure their well-being is to help them maintain caring and loving relationships with both parents. Don't place your children in the middle, and don't use them as instruments for venting your anger toward your partner. Try to minimize the disruption in your children's lives and help them anticipate what changes are inevitable and how you intend to help them adjust to these changes. Explanations about why you're separating or divorcing should be respectful of each partner and tailored to your child's age and ability to deal with complicated relationship issues.

Children often feel powerless and vulnerable during and following a divorce. They worry about where they'll live, where they'll go to school, whether they'll have to give up their friends and make new ones, how often they'll get to see each parent, whether they'll be separated from their siblings, and whether their economic quality of life will be reduced— whether that involves the car a youngster was hoping for when turning 16 or the opportunity to attend the college of his or her choice. Younger children are particularly vulnerable to fears of being abandoned. Children of any age are susceptible to feeling guilty or responsible for their parents' divorce. They're also likely to feel angry—either because of the negative impact on their own lives or, especially among older children, from a moral perspective and wish that somehow their parents would have "done better." It's not uncommon to see signs of anxiety (for example, tearfulness or difficulties with sleeping), anger (for example, temper tantrums and verbal or physical aggression toward others), withdrawal or clinginess, or rebellion against parental rules. It's also not uncommon for anger to be expressed more openly toward the custodial parent, in part because that relationship may be seen by the child as safer and more secure.

Consider letting neighbors or the parents of your children's best friends know about your separation or divorce; they may be able to provide your children some relief or stability when things are particularly chaotic for you and your partner. You may also want to inform your children's teachers, particularly if a child has experienced a recent increase in school-related problems.

Offer your children an opportunity to talk about their feelings and listen without judgment. Offer encouragement and reassurance that, with time and effort, things will improve and become more stable. Most of all, remember that a critical factor in your children's adjustment following a divorce will be how well you and your former partner collaborate in taking care of and making decisions about your children.

How Should I Care for Myself?

In many ways, the emotional effects of separation or divorce for adult partners are similar to those for their children. You may feel powerless and vulnerable and may worry about where you'll live, how much money you'll have, how often you'll see your children, whether your family or friends will desert you, and whether you'll find a new partner. You may feel abandoned or rejected by your partner. You may feel profoundly guilty for ending your relationship or causing your partner to end it. Anxiety and depression are common effects of divorce and may result in difficulties in sleeping, concentrating at work, or taking care of yourself such as by sticking to good nutrition and exercise.

Preparing for separation and divorce by working through the logistics ahead of time, and by strengthening social and emotional support from friends and family, can keep these negative reactions from becoming too severe or lasting too long. Time may not heal all wounds, but it helps. Review the important aspects of self-care described in Chapter 5. In what ways are you already not caring for yourself? Some aspects of self-care may become less available when you end your relationship—for example, making time to exercise or eat healthy meals. Will you lose some of your opportunities to socialize with couple friends or with members of your partner's family? Will you be less comfortable or feel less welcome in your church or synagogue? Try to anticipate how you could offset some of these losses—for example, by pursuing interests or activities that you've neglected previously or by developing new hobbies or beginning new exercise routines that you've put off. Try to remember that in addition to marking the end of a relationship, divorce symbolizes a new beginning. Beyond the initial grieving, separation or divorce can provide opportunity for growth and renewal.

Connie and Jared struggled for a year to make sense of Jared's affair. Both in their early 40s, they had married somewhat later in life and had no children. Jared's brief affair was with an 18-year-old who rented an apartment in a duplex he had owned since he was single. Shortly after Connie learned of his affair, she moved into an apartment of her own and tried to regain an emotional foothold in her life.

Both partners wanted to save their marriage, if possible, and agreed to marriage counseling. Connie and Jared shed many tears in the early sessions—Connie from her deep hurt, and Jared from his equally deep remorse. Even from the beginning, they continued to support each other in their respective small retail businesses while living separately. In exploring the context for Jared's affair, they both gained insight into Jared's lifelong pattern of seeking out situations that provided excitement while risking his own welfare. By engaging in his affair, Jared had risked not only his own well-being, but Connie's too.

Jared developed a better understanding of his childhood experiences that had contributed to his pattern of risky behaviors and poor judgment. Over several months he took important steps to restrain his behaviors—not only when he was interacting with other people, but also in his own private life. He continued to work faithfully at supporting Connie and regaining her trust. But Jared also struggled with his own mixed feelings about marriage. He loved Connie and didn't want their relationship to end, but the confines of marriage at times felt like more than he had bargained for. Being able to go when and where he pleased had been a part of his single life he hadn't realized he would miss.

After months of examining and challenging her own feelings, Connie concluded that although she would always care for Jared and regard him as a friend, she could never regain the depth of intimacy or admiration for him that she viewed as essential for a healthy marriage. She understood that Jared might be able to adjust to boundaries that were vital to her, but she wanted a partner who prized her and aspired to the same vision of marriage she had—not someone who would labor to accommodate it. Following several more months of struggling over what to do, they tearfully decided to end their marriage and move on separately.

Connie and Jared continued to support each other in carrying out this decision. They kept helping out in each other's business, while also developing new personal relationships. Within the following two years, both Connie and Jared had each found a new romantic partner. Although their interactions gradually diminished, they remained friends.

What If I Still Can't Make Up My Mind?

After carefully evaluating all of these factors related to moving forward, you may still have difficulty making a decision. **Common situations leading to continued indecision include the following:**

- Your partner has undertaken important changes, but there are still too many unresolved issues for you to feel confident that your marriage can work in the long run.
- Your partner continues to behave in ways that interfere with restoring trust or intimacy, but these haven't yet convinced you that the only remaining course is to move on separately.

- Your partner has done everything you've asked and you've let go of your deep hurt and anger, but you haven't recovered feelings of intimacy and aren't sure they'll ever come back.
- Your relationship isn't so bad that you can't tolerate it, and you're reluctant to end it because of the negative effects you believe this would have on your children.

Resolving the first two problems may require obtaining additional information and engaging your partner in the process. If your partner has made *some* but limited progress, for example, talk with your partner to point out the significant gains you've made and your hopefulness based on this, but also pinpoint lingering concerns and explore what you could each do to resolve them. If your partner is still putting your relationship at risk, confront him with the behaviors that are blocking recovery from the affair and be clear about what steps will have to be taken for you to stay in the relationship. In both cases, consider a time line for achieving further progress and reevaluating the situation to determine whether you can reach a clearer decision about how to move forward.

If your partner is already doing everything you've asked to restore a close relationship but you remain stuck emotionally, your efforts may need to focus more on you and your own barriers to moving on. In most cases of this sort, we recommend staying in the marriage and continuing to work toward a caring relationship to see whether feelings of intimacy return. The trauma of an affair often produces a kind of emotional numbness, and people vary in how long they take to recover their feelings. Two caveats: First, it's important to develop a reasonable time line for your feelings to return. Even with consistent effort, it may take months or even years for feelings of emotional closeness to return; no one can tell you how long is long enough to see if those feelings come back. Second, note our emphasis on continued effort. Simply waiting for intimate feelings to return on their own, without actively working toward promoting emotional and physical closeness, is almost destined to fail.

Finally, if you're stuck because of concern over the potential effects on your children, consider talking to trusted friends who have gone through divorce with children of ages similar to those of yours. Reading reputable books written from a variety of perspectives may give you a balanced understanding of children's vulnerability and resilience to their parents' divorce. Consulting with a mental health professional experienced in family processes and children's development can also tell you more about common reactions to separation or divorce and how these may or may not apply to your own children.

It's important not to rush into decisions or act on initial impulses before you're confident that you've considered all the relevant factors to a reasonable degree. It's also important to consider which actions are sustainable or reversible. For example, deciding to stay in the marriage for three months to collect more information may be less disruptive than separating temporarily to evaluate what that's like. It's also important, however, not to delay your decision indefinitely. Maintaining the status quo by avoiding a decision altogether rarely makes the current situation better.

What's Next?

Work through the following exercises, which will help you evaluate factors involved in reaching an explicit decision about how to move forward and then examine how to implement your decision. If you've decided to move forward by staying in this relationship, the second exercise will help you examine some remaining tasks aimed at promoting healing from the affair and strengthening your relationship—including issues of rebuilding trust. If instead you've decided to pursue separation or divorce, that exercise will help you think through specific things you'll need to anticipate and plan for—including the initial transition as well as the longer term.

After you've worked through these exercises, Chapter 14 will help you step back and gain perspective on all you've worked toward and learned since the affair, as well as what to anticipate in the coming months.

——————————— Exercises ———————————

EXERCISE 13.1.
REACHING A DECISION ABOUT HOW TO MOVE FORWARD

Whether to continue or end your current relationship is a huge decision. If you haven't yet decided what to do, this exercise may help you reach that decision. If you've already decided how to move forward, this exercise will help clarify the factors that went into your decision.

Make two lists—one recording reasons to move on together and the other including reasons to move on separately. Consider factors you identified previously in working through the exercises for Chapters 7 to 10: aspects of the partner who had the affair, aspects of the injured partner, your relationship, and outside influences. Not all factors are likely to be equally important, so it can also be helpful to assign numbers or weights to each of the items on your list—for example, 3 for very important, 2 for somewhat important, and 1 for least important.

For instance, one very important reason for staying together in your relationship might be:

"My partner is truly sorry about what she did, and she's acknowledged many things about herself that made her vulnerable. I can see the changes she's making. I love her very much, and if she continues to work at change, I want to work hard as well at making our relationship succeed."

Or you might believe that a somewhat important reason to stay together is:

"The reality is that ending this relationship would leave me in a pretty tough place financially. I haven't worked outside the home for quite a while, and I'm not sure I could get a job to support myself. That may not sound like the best reason to stay in a marriage, but it's something I need to consider."

Alternatively, you might decide that an important reason to move on separately is:

"Although we've generally gotten along well for most of our marriage, I think in large part we were staying together from a fear of being alone. We've tried hard, but I don't think there's 'real love' between us. I don't want to sound like a naive romantic, but I believe I could develop a much more loving and fulfilling relationship with someone else."

Once you've completed your lists and rated the importance of these different factors, pull this information together and see where it leads you. We don't propose you simply add up the values and see whether staying versus leaving got more points. This decision isn't a simple mathematical process, nor is it just a matter of reason or logic. The best decisions are those that combine your reason and logic along with your feelings or emotions. If your reason tells you one thing and your emotions tell you something else, that's okay. Keep working, and eventually your mind and your heart may line up with each other.

Be sure you give yourself time to work through this process. After identifying and evaluating factors in your decision, come back to your notes again a few days or weeks later. Reconsider your evaluations not only at times when you're feeling distressed in your relationship, but also when you're feeling more optimistic. That way, you're more likely to arrive at a balanced view that considers all the relevant factors and emphasizes those that you've determined to be most important.

If you and your partner are both reading this book, complete this exercise independently and then talk about where you both are in your decision. You may want to talk with each other after you first make the lists and consider what you might want to do. If you're both leaning the same way, good—but still take time to consider your decision further.

If you're moving in different directions, this will likely lead to very difficult conversations. Listen to, and try to respect, your partner's perspective, using the communication skills you've learned. Remember that understanding your partner's perspective doesn't mean agreeing with it. You're entitled to your own opinion and decision no matter what your partner thinks or how painful it might be to implement. If you aren't ready to talk with your partner after you first complete your lists, that's okay. Take your time to think through these critical issues before initiating the discussion, but be sure to talk with your partner before reaching a final decision.

If you're reading this book alone, complete the exercise and try to get your partner to do the same. Even without reading the book or working through previous exercises, your partner may be able to list some pros and cons of staying in the relationship versus ending it. If your partner won't participate in this exercise at any level, do it alone and talk with your partner about the decision you're contemplating.

As you complete this exercise, you also may discover that you would benefit from talking with a mental health professional or trusted spiritual adviser. If so, review the guidelines presented in Chapter 5 regarding considerations in seeking additional outside assistance.

EXERCISE 13.2. IMPLEMENTING YOUR DECISION TO STAY OR GO

If Moving Forward Together

If you've decided to move forward together in your relationship, make a list of the things you need to address to give your relationship the best chance of succeeding in the future. Focus on changes that each of you would need to make as individuals, changes for your relationship, and changes in relating to others around you. Take your time on this list. *After listing important changes in these areas, talk with each other about specific strategies for implementing these changes.* Review your responses to exercises for Chapters 7 through 10. Hold yourselves and each other accountable for the decisions you make regarding steps toward change.

You also may decide to do something symbolic to demonstrate this new phase in your relationship—for example, having a public or private rededication ceremony. In that ceremony, make your vows personal and real. If rededicating yourselves in a private ceremony, you might want to hold the list of changes you've agreed to in your hand—not just committing to each other in general terms, but also committing to specific actions that you've identified as vital to your relationship. Whether you do something symbolic or not, make yourselves and each other accountable for following through. Review your list and the steps you've each taken a month from now, and then again six months later.

If Moving Forward Separately

If you've decided to move forward by ending your relationship, how will you do that in the healthiest way possible? In ending the relationship, you'll need to address both emotional and practical issues. *Your feelings will evolve over time, so agree to have several conversations with your partner about the feelings you're both having and how they change.* It's often necessary to address some of the emotional issues first before moving on to pragmatic issues. In discussing emotional issues, try to be as honest and caring as possible and maintain a balance in what you share. Don't just focus on your hurtful or angry feelings. Relationships are often hard to end because you're giving up a lot of good things. We've worked with couples who, while ending their marriage, talked with each other about the good they experienced from their relationship—what they learned, how they grew, and what they'll miss. Those couples moved on better than others who ended their relationships in anger.

Some major practical issues include concerns related to living arrangements, finances, division of property, and informing others. Other important issues may include how to care for your children and how to care for yourself. *Make a list of the important practical issues you'll need to address.* Although at times it may be difficult for you and your partner to have constructive conversations about these critical issues, treating each other with dignity and fairness will leave each of you feeling better about the other and yourself. *Write down what you need to do to make this process productive and respectful.* For example, you may decide that it's best to discuss these issues only on weekends, when you're both feeling rested. You might agree to address only one issue during a conversation so emotions don't build. Or you may decide that you want a mediator or mental health professional to help you with discussions if they become too volatile when the two of you have these conversations alone.

14

What Lies Ahead?

Miriam had been trying to listen to her friend, Nina, but her mind kept wandering. "I'm totally lost," Nina despaired. "It's a nightmare, and I wish I could just wake up and find it all gone." A few weeks earlier Nina had discovered that her husband of 11 years, Tony, had been having an affair for six months with a woman he met while coaching their son's soccer team. Nina and Tony were now living in separate rooms of their house; their 9-year-old son and 5-year-old daughter sensed the deep tension between their parents but said little. Miriam's daughter and Nina's daughter were best friends, and Miriam had seen her daughter's friend collapsing in tears at the slightest frustration. Nina now seemed on the verge of tears as well.

"I just don't know what to do," Miriam heard Nina continue. "Tony doesn't seem to be able to make up his mind. I don't think he's sleeping with her anymore, but I know they talk almost every day. I don't want to lose Tony, but I can't imagine ever getting over this. We have two children to care for. We're close to each other's family. We had dreams together—everything to live for, everything to lose. How could he have done this?"

Miriam debated how much to share with her friend. She and Jesse had been through a similar crisis two years earlier, following Miriam's own affair. Her affair had been shorter and with someone from out of state she met at a business convention. But the effects had been just as devastating. Nina didn't know about Miriam's affair—but Miriam certainly knew about the trauma that Nina was experiencing. She re-

called how close she and Jesse had come to ending their marriage, and how hard they had each struggled to hold on to their relationship and rebuild it from scratch. It had taken three months before their shouting matches finally ended, and another six months before they had any real understanding of what had happened and why. Now, two years later, they knew they had survived the worst part. There were still heartaches that came each time either one of them remembered Miriam's affair. But they were stronger and wiser now. They had renewed their commitment to each other and understood better than ever what that required of them.

Miriam knew that Nina and her husband would need more help than she or Jesse could provide. But at least she could offer some understanding of Nina's feelings and encouragement about their potential to recover. "It's a long and difficult process," Miriam spoke softly. "But I think I can tell you about what it might look like . . . "

What lies ahead, and how can you prepare for it? Like Miriam or her husband, Jesse, you may still struggle at times with painful memories of the affair. We hope that you've also gained strength and wisdom from working through the previous chapters and have a clearer vision of how you want to move forward—either separately or with your partner. In this final chapter, we'll help you anticipate what still lies ahead. For most people, recovery from an affair continues even after they've reached decisions about how to move on. Whether with or without your current partner, knowing what challenges may arise and having some strategies for managing them can help with continuing the recovery process.

>>> **Safeguarding your current or future relationship and moving forward in a healthy way requires that you:**
- **Anticipate setbacks involving hurt feelings and painful memories.**
- **Use your memories of the previous affair to prevent any recurrences.**
- **Avoid situations and people who place your relationship at risk.**
- **Use the communication skills you've gained to:**
  - **Express your feelings more constructively.**
  - **Manage conflict and reach decisions together more effectively.**

- **Promote physical closeness.**
- **Prize your relationship.**
- **Stay focused on your vision for the future.**
- **Seek out additional help you may need for yourself or your relationship.**

Anticipate Setbacks

Either you or your partner may continue to experience hurtful feelings or memories related to the affair. We hope that with time and effort these will become increasingly less frequent, less intense, and briefer in terms of their hurtful impact. Injured partners tend to struggle with hurtful memories longer than participating partners (although the opposite sometimes occurs). Some circumstances—for example, anniversaries of events related to the affair or special occasions in your own relationship—may stir up memories of the affair that have been quiet for weeks or months. Hurtful recollections of the affair don't necessarily indicate "going backward," "losing ground," or "starting all over again." Instead, they're more often a painful but natural part of the process of moving forward.

Anticipating setbacks and placing them in perspective can help prevent them from becoming traumatic occasions in themselves. You can use the skills you developed in Chapter 2 for dealing with flashbacks. For example, if you're the one struggling with hurtful memories, you can decide to cope with these on your own using self-care techniques, or you can share your struggles with your partner and request separate time for yourself or special time together as a way of experiencing closeness and reassurance. If you recognize that your partner is struggling with memories from the affair, you can offer acceptance of your partner's feelings, ask your partner what you could do right then that would be most helpful, reaffirm the progress you've already achieved as a couple, and reassure your partner that you'll continue to be there to move forward together as best you both can.

Make Good Use of Your Memories

Use your memories of the affair as a way of "keeping watch" or remaining vigilant—not in a fearful way, but in a healthy, protective way. Once an affair occurs, the illusion that many couples have that "it could never happen to us" has been shattered. Moving forward in a constructive way requires continuing to use what you've learned from the affair to keep you and your relationship safe. For example, if your marriage became vulnerable to an affair because you or your partner were devoting too much time to work or to others, have you begun to slip back into that unhealthy pattern? If the affair served as a "wake-up call" and led to increased caring and patience you offered to one another, have you since let your guard down and started to take each other for granted? It's important not to lose the emotional closeness or intensity of renewed commitment that the affair may have brought about.

You can also use your memories of the affair constructively if you've decided to move on separately from your partner. For example, you may have a better understanding of what's most important to you in considering a new relationship. You may understand yourself at a deeper level and know better how to build and maintain a relationship that is less vulnerable to an affair. You may also be better prepared to recognize outside risks and know how to address them.

Viewed from this perspective, memories of the affair can be something other than just hurtful or disruptive. At an appropriate level, they can serve as a useful reminder of how to move forward in a more thoughtful and purposeful way, keeping your values and priorities in clear order.

Avoid Unnecessary Risks

No one else has as much at stake in your marriage as you do. No one else will likely work as hard to protect your marriage as you must. Employers often demand your increased effort. Community organizations plead for your time. Children present endless needs for your time and emotional energy. Friends may ask you to socialize separately with them. Outsiders in pursuit of a relationship may minimize the importance of marriage and family commitments you already have. *The world is full of risks and threats to your marriage.*

You need to take charge in actively avoiding people or situations that, either directly or indirectly, place your marriage at increased vulnerability to an affair. Outsiders don't need to encourage infidelity to place your marriage at increased risk. They simply need to encourage your involvement in a relationship or in activities that don't honor your marriage as your first priority. It's up to you to resist these outside influences.

Keep Communicating

Talk often and well. Common factors contributing to an affair involve emotional distance that sets in when partners start to lead parallel but disengaged lives or when resentments accumulate from ineffective strategies for dealing with conflict or reaching decisions together. Recovery from an affair forces partners to talk with each other. They have to find ways of expressing and understanding the feelings triggered by the affair. They need to reach decisions about how to survive the initial chaos as well as longer-range decisions about how to move forward. However, too often after the initial turmoil has subsided, couples slip back into previous communication patterns that interfered with collaboration and emotional closeness.

There are two ways of maintaining effective communication. One involves daily "connection talks" of 10 to 15 minutes as a way of learning about what's going on in each other's life. Resist the temptation to reduce your exchanges to "How was your day?" followed by "Fine" or a similarly brief reply. Use open-ended prompts such as "Tell me about your day. What was the best part? What was the most frustrating part?" Create a time to have this discussion when you can actually listen to each other. If you wait for talk time to appear on its own, it probably won't. You have to make the time and effort to stay connected. No day should end without at least a 10- to 15-minute reconnection set apart from other interactions and symbolizing the importance you place on your relationship.

An additional way of maintaining effective communication is to set aside one 20- to 30-minute time each week when you check in with each other regarding relationship issues. The goal of this exchange is to ensure that any issues that have developed during the week are recognized by each of you and have either been addressed already or have been identified as needing further discussion. This exchange can begin with the simple question "How are we doing?" This permits you to talk about things you've done well and ways in which you've felt close, as well as identifying any concerns you have. If the relationship has been going well, discuss why or how that's so. What did you most appreciate this past week? When did you feel closest? When did you and your partner resolve a difference or reach a decision together in ways that affirmed your collaboration? You can also use this time to discuss what's coming up in the days or week ahead that will require your working together.

Keep Touching

Work at staying physically connected. Use hugs or gentle touches throughout the day—when you first wake up, when you pass one another or work side by side, and before you go to sleep. Hold hands when sitting together on the couch or going for walks. Snuggle often. Physical closeness between partners helps to ease tensions or minor irritations that can arise from within or outside the relationship.

Make time for lovemaking. If you or your partner struggle with one or more sexual difficulties, as discussed in Chapter 7, seek professional help. Talk with each other about ways to maintain or revitalize your sexual relationship. Remember that it's not necessary or realistic to experience "great sex" every time you and your partner are intimate. What's important is that you stay physically connected in ways that feel mutually caring.

Prize Your Relationship

Prizing your relationship goes beyond protecting against risks and maintaining good communication. It involves bringing to your relationship a level of energy and commitment that nurtures and strengthens your bond. Look for opportunities to be together in new and exciting ways. Think of each other during the day and find ways of expressing this to your partner—for example, by a brief phone call that begins, "I was just thinking about you and wanted you to know that," or by a love note left for your partner to discover during the day. Think back to the best times of your relationship when you felt most special—perhaps to your initial courtship or times later in the marriage when you felt a special connection between you. What did you each say and do that let the other one feel cherished? Did you set aside time for each other even when there were pressing demands from outside? Prizing each other requires resisting the temptation to take each other for granted. It requires some imagination and creativity, supported by enduring commitment.

Stay Focused on Your Vision

There are two kinds of thinking that get couples into trouble. The first involves adopting a wait-and-see attitude. Individuals adopting this attitude create an uncertainty in themselves and in their partners. They communicate—explicitly or implicitly—"Things are okay for now, but you never know about the future. I'm here for the time being, but I'm making no guarantees because anything could happen." Waiting for something bad to happen gets in the way of making good things happen. Eventually, in most relationships, bad things *do* happen at one level or another. They're more likely to happen if there's a void left in the marriage because one or both partners are holding back to see what develops before committing to a vision for the future; moreover, the impact of negative events is greater because there isn't a strong foundation of continued positive interactions to help offset or cushion them.

The second kind of thinking that gets couples into trouble is the throwing-in-the-towel attitude during times of conflict. Following an affair, some couples restore a fragile alliance but don't do the daily work to make things solid between them. Their marriage remains vulnerable to the least stressor and easily gets thrown into a tailspin. Minor disagreements rapidly escalate into major conflicts, and either partner may threaten divorce. Threats of ending the relationship have a destructive impact that lasts well beyond the situation in which they're made—even when partners later apologize and "take back" what they've said.

Resist the temptation to make such threats, no matter how hurt or angry you feel in the moment. The best way to resist despair and impulses to "give up" is to keep a clear vision of how far you've come and where you want to end up. It's okay to get blown off course, so long as you know where you're headed and can reset your direction. Sometimes that requires saying to yourself, "This feels pretty awful right now, but we've been through worse and survived it. The way we've gotten back on course in the past is to stop doing further damage, evaluate what's gone wrong, and then figure out how to take the next step forward. I need to separate what I'm feeling in this moment from what I know we're committed to in the longer view."

Seek Out Additional Help If Needed

Recovery from an affair is rarely a smooth process. The learning and practice of new skills required to move forward rarely occur all at once. You should anticipate going back and rereading chapters of this book as you move forward. Previous issues will reemerge—sometimes in their original form, sometimes in a slightly new form. New issues will emerge as well, but many of these can be addressed by using the resources that you've already developed by working through the previous chapters.

It's not necessary or even desirable that you work through recovery on your own. If you and your partner have decided to move on together, it's important that you draw on each other for comfort and strength as you struggle forward. You'll need to be patient with one another when reexperiencing hurt feelings—offering both acceptance and encouragement. You may also draw on the support of your closest friends with whom you've shared information about your struggles. Having someone who supports your marriage during your most difficult struggles can be vital when wrestling with waves of panic or anger from the affair or when working hard to maintain firm boundaries against outside influences or people who threaten your commitment to fidelity.

It's sometimes important to seek out assistance from those with special expertise in recovering from relationship wounds. Clergy can often provide a spiritual perspective that promotes comfort, strength, and healing. You or your partner may also benefit from talking with a mental health professional—either separately or together—to deal with the special challenges you're continuing to face in moving forward. You may find it useful to read through portions of Chapter 5 again regarding considerations in seeking additional outside assistance.

Final Words

In our own experience as therapists, we've never stopped admiring the deep values and profound commitment shown by individuals and couples who have approached us for help in making the right decisions following an affair. Their openness in baring their wounds and genuineness in seeking help in moving forward have been testaments to their strength. We've often been more confident of their ability to reach and implement healthy decisions about moving forward than they have, and we've rarely been disappointed.

In our final words to you, we want to voice our confidence in your ability to make the right decisions in your own life about how to move forward from this affair. We don't underestimate how difficult this struggle will be. We know that there may be times when you continue to feel hurt, angry, sad, anxious, or even hopeless. We also know that, by working through the chapters and exercises we've offered here, you've already shown a level of commitment that distinguishes you from others who give up early on or rush to a "quick fix" without doing the hard work of figuring out what went wrong and then embracing a more complete and more difficult rebuilding process.

You can do this. We know this from our experience of watching hundreds of others do what first seemed impossible. We want you to know that *you* can do this as well. You're not alone. Be patient, be persistent, and be strong. Most important, hold on to hope. You've already survived the worst. We're confident that you can now create the best.

Additional Resources

Strengthening Your Marriage

Christensen, A., & Jacobson, N. S. (1999). *Reconcilable differences*. New York: Guilford Press.

Doherty, W. J. (2001). *Take back your marriage: Sticking together in a world that pulls us apart*. New York: Guilford Press.

Gottman, J. M. (1999). *The seven principles for making marriage work*. New York: Three Rivers Press.

Enright, R. D. (2001). *Forgiveness is a choice: A step-by-step process for resolving anger and restoring hope*. Washington, DC: American Psychological Association.

Dealing with Specific Problem Areas (Sex, Money, and Children)

McCarthy, B., & McCarthy, E. (2003). *Rekindling desire: A step-by-step program to help low-sex and no-sex marriages*. New York: Brunner-Routledge.

Liberman, G., & Lavine, A. (1998). *Love, marriage and money: Understanding and achieving financial compatibility before—and after—you say "I do."* Chicago: Dearborn Financial Publishing.

Dinkmeyer, D., McKay, G. D., & Dinkmeyer, D. (1997). *The parent's handbook: Systematic training for effective parenting (STEP)*. Circle Pines, MN: American Guidance Service.

Sells, S. P. (2001). *Parenting your out-of-control teenager: 7 steps to reestablish authority and reclaim love*. New York: St. Martin's Press.

Approaching Divorce

Kirshenbaum, M. (1996). *Too good to leave, too bad to stay: A step-by-step guide to help you decide whether to stay in or get out of your relationship.* New York: Plume.

Ahrons, C. (1994). *The good divorce: Keeping your family together when your marriage comes apart.* New York: HarperCollins.

Wallerstein, J. S., & Blakeslee, S. (2003). *What about the kids? Raising your children before, during, and after divorce.* New York: Hyperion.

Finding a Therapist Near You

American Psychological Association
locator.apahelpcenter.org

American Association for Marriage and Family Therapy
therapistlocator.net

Australian Psychological Society
www.psychology.org.au/psych/referral_service/Default.aspx

British Psychological Society
www.bps.org.uk/e-services/find-a-psychologist/psychoindex.cfm

Index

About the Authors

Douglas K. Snyder, PhD, is Professor of Psychology and Director of Clinical Training at Texas A&M University. He received the American Psychological Association's award for Distinguished Contributions to Family Psychology for his research on marital satisfaction and therapy. His edited books include *Treating Difficult Couples* (Guilford Press) and *Emotion Regulation in Couples and Families* (American Psychological Association). He lives in College Station, Texas, where he also engages in private practice.

Donald H. Baucom, PhD, is Professor of Psychology at the University of North Carolina–Chapel Hill. His research, funded in part by the National Institutes of Health, focuses on couples and marriage. His six books about couples include his widely used text coauthored with Norman Epstein, *Enhanced Cognitive-Behavioral Therapy for Couples* (American Psychological Association). He lives in Chapel Hill, North Carolina, and was ranked as one of the top marital therapists and researchers in the United States by *Good Housekeeping*'s national survey of mental health professionals.

Kristina Coop Gordon, PhD, is Associate Professor of Clinical Psychology at the University of Tennessee. Her research focuses on forgiveness, infidelity, and couple therapy. In addition to her academic work, she maintains a private practice in Knoxville, Tennessee, where she resides.